Spiritual Awakening

Learn Reiki Self Healing, and Improve Your Energy Level

(Try the Reiki With Crystals to Improve Your Spiritual Life and to Reduce Some Ailments)

Walter Bevell

Published by Rob Miles

Walter Bevell

All Rights Reserved

Spiritual Awakening: Learn Reiki Self Healing, and Improve Your Energy Level (Try the Reiki With Crystals to Improve Your Spiritual Life and to Reduce Some Ailments)

ISBN 978-1-989990-51-3

All rights reserved. No part of this guide may be reproduced in any form without permission in writing from the publisher except in the case of brief quotations embodied in critical articles or reviews.

Legal & Disclaimer

The information contained in this book is not designed to replace or take the place of any form of medicine or professional medical advice. The information in this book has been provided for educational and entertainment purposes only.

The information contained in this book has been compiled from sources deemed reliable, and it is accurate to the best of the Author's knowledge; however, the Author cannot guarantee its accuracy and validity and cannot be held liable for any errors or omissions. Changes are periodically made to this book. You must consult your doctor or get professional medical advice before using any of the suggested remedies, techniques, or information in this book.

Upon using the information contained in this book, you agree to hold harmless the Author from and against any damages, costs, and expenses, including any legal fees potentially resulting from the application of any of the information provided by this guide. This disclaimer applies to any damages or injury caused by the use and application, whether directly or indirectly, of any advice or information presented, whether for breach of contract, tort, negligence, personal injury, criminal intent, or under any other cause of action.

You agree to accept all risks of using the information presented inside this book. You need to consult a professional medical practitioner in order to ensure you are both able and healthy enough to participate in this program.

Table of Contents

INTRODUCTION 1

CHAPTER 1: HEALING MEDITATION - YOUR GUIDE TO BALANCING THE CHAKRAS 2

CHAPTER 2: THE CURRENT STATE OF REIKI TRAINING 26

CHAPTER 3: THE ROOT CHAKRA 32

CHAPTER 4: THE THREE PILLARS OF REIKI 38

CHAPTER 5: BODY ENERGY SYSTEMS 47

CHAPTER 6: BASIC YOGA POSTURES 56

CHAPTER 7: THE REIKI ATTUNEMENTS. 68

CHAPTER 8: SYMBOLS AND ATTUNEMENTS 75

CHAPTER 9: CONSIDERING REIKI FOR HEALTH 101

CHAPTER 10: THE CHAKRAS AND THE ENERGY BODY 104

CHAPTER 11: THE FOURTH CHAKRA 112

CHAPTER 12: CIRCLES MEDITATION 116

CHAPTER 13: HANDS ON HEALING" IN RELIGION 123

CHAPTER 14: ADDITIONAL HEALING TECHNIQUES (ADVANCED STUDENTS ONLY).. 127

CHAPTER 15: EVERYDAY REIKI 150

CHAPTER 16: MORE POSES FOR BEGINNERS.................. 157

CHAPTER 17: REIKI FAQS 164

CHAPTER 18: LIVING A KIND AND COMPASSIONATE LIFE 168

CHAPTER 19: THE 5 PRINCIPLES OF REIKI....................... 183

CHAPTER 20: EXPLAINING DISTANT REIKI...................... 199

CONCLUSION.. 203

Introduction

This book contains proven steps and strategies on how to better understand the way Reiki healing can help you live a happier and healthier life. I hope that, through this book, you will appreciate how Reiki can be a wonderful blessing that can alter your whole life for the better. When you finally decide to become a Reiki practitioner, you will be openly linked to a potent and divine source of healing energy that can help you become free from the stress, pains, and suffering you are going through.

Thanks again for downloading this book, I hope you enjoy it!

Chapter 1: Healing Meditation - Your Guide To Balancing The Chakras

Do you accept that upbeat and positive considerations can cause recuperating? This is because of the way that your body and mind will pursue to your musings. If your contemplations go a different way, will likewise encounter a negative change. With such, you will come to understand that Meditation as an amending procedure can incredibly help in giving wellbeing.

Adjusting Chakras

Fundamentally, your body condition can be in a decent state when you consider beneficial things. Along these lines, when you fill your brain with negative contemplations, something very similar pursues. This is how your body can impact the Chakras. It very well may be either through direct messages, through immediate considerations that we select to go into.

The otherworldly body isn't quite the same as the physical body. For example, if you expend unhealthy nourishment, this will bring about getting to be overweight and experience the ill effects of different infirmities like diabetes, hypertension, and others. When your musings are negative, the body atmosphere takes in all these similarly that your body retains sustenance. Like the physical body, the air cannot figure out what is awful and bravo. What it does is that it ingests what is accessible at a specific time and utilizes it — because of this, adjusting Chakras through Meditation is extremely basic.

Mostly, when you convey a negative idea and spotlight on it, you can have the coordinating Chakra to accompany a negative inclination to the remaining

Chakras. This makes the entire Chakra framework to destabilize. The side effects of this marvel bring about physical diseases, negative feelings; just as relationship troubles. Subsequently, making an equalization on the Chakras through Meditation can be your underlying step towards mental, profound, physical, and passionate prosperity.

Steps in Healing Meditation

Acquiring amicability can be your initial step, to begin with, the recuperating procedure. These Meditation steps can help you in adjusting your Chakras and investigating or opening a progressively specific recuperating practice:

Ensure that you are sitting in a spot that is tranquil, protected, and loaded up with nonpartisan vitality. Wear agreeable garments.

Choose the best position for you. You can either sit on a seat or the floor with your legs crossed.

Close eyes and stay concentrated on your relaxing. Ensure that your breaths are originating from the outline and let muscles relax each time you rest.

Continue with Meditation and spotlight on your Chakras. Consider it a streaming light while turning it clockwise and turning it out on the other heading at that point, pulling it in once more.

Do this with the remainder of your body Chakras. Take in full breaths and open your eyes gradually.

By thinking about these steps in Meditation, you will, without a doubt, feel relaxed, quiet, focused, and free from certain body diseases.

Balance Your Chakras With Acupressure

Holistic healers have united the old intelligence of both Chinese and Indian prescription by utilizing needle therapy related to adjusting the chakras, which supports physical, passionate, and otherworldly wellbeing. A minor departure from this is to adapt your chakras using acupressure and essential oils.

Acupressure, as the name recommends, substitutes applying weight to the essential purposes of the body as opposed to utilizing needles, as in the exemplary routine with regards to conventional needle therapy.

Various investigations show some extremely profitable employments of acupressure.

One examination proposed that treatment with the Tapas Acupressure Technique, for instance, can help individuals recoup and keep up their wellbeing and working. Acupressure may help with queasiness, while another examination found that it might be more compelling than the most acclaimed back rub treatment of all, Swedish back rub. Utilizing fragrant essential oils gets the intensity of fragrance based treatment to supplement the customary Chinese and Indian holistic cures.

The ideas fundamental the utilization of acupressure to rebalance the seven head chakras are nearly equivalent to in needle therapy. The thing that matters is that touch replaces the addition of needle therapy needles at the pertinent "acupoints." These focuses are extensively equal to the seven chakras portrayed in the Indian mending reasoning.

In fragrance based treatment, various scents are related to multiple characteristics and resonances, or vibrations of vitality. They can be utilized on any piece of the body or discharged into the air, where they neutralize the pheromones that individuals radiate, particularly in distressing circumstances.

The thought behind utilizing fragrant healing pair with acupressure is that adequacy is commonly improved by coordinating the forces and properties of specific oils to the distinctive strength focuses that are spoken to by the seven chakras. These are situated along the midline of the body, relating with focuses along the spine, from the head to the crotch. The word chakra signifies 'wheel' yet in Hinduism and Buddhism the chakras are additionally imagined as blooms that can be opened like a bloom - for this situation, using fragrant oils.

Various professionals may suggest multiple oils, or various mixes of oils, for use on the distinctive chakras. For instance, the third chakra is related to the stomach similar tract. Like this holistic healers will choose an essential oil that is accepted to follow up on the stomach related framework, for example, peppermint oil. Utilizing oils and acupressure together is a method for 'bending over' on the adequacy of the treatment.

Acupressure with essential oils can rebalance your chakras, discharging the progression of yin and yang by cooperating to coordinate personality, body, and soul.

The Chakras and Energy Streams

Chakras allude to the energy focuses that are related to the sensory system. Each chakra in the body has a specific vibration associated with one of the shades of the range. The chakra takes in the shading energy from the aura that envelopes the body. Different hues are allocated to their separate power focuses, which are situated inside the spine.

Seven chakras make up the body, filling in as the fundamental supervisors of energies that go all through the body. Regardless of whether the chakras are not physically noticeable in the body, they are identified with the fields of energy that encompass the body. To help in making the energy of the chakras adjusted, the Chakra Jewelry and Chakra Light Catchers have been made.

Chakras invigorate the physical body and are identified with the collaborations of the psyche and body. These energy focuses are viewed as loci of prana or life energy that stream along the nadis or pathways.

A stream of energy enters the body in the chakras. A similar energy stream saturates the universe, the divinities, and the "unpretentious bodies." The Nadis, which are spoken to as veins, nerves, and cylinders in the Indian custom, associate the distinctive chakras. There are a vast number of chakras. The channels are identified with excellent harmonies so the accompanying can be made: hues, geometry, components, and streams of energy, among others.

At the point when two people participate in sex, the lights from their sex chakras are consolidated. At that point, the purple light waves make figures, whose beauty relies upon the sort and power of affection between the two accomplices. When two individuals genuinely adore one another, they make an incredible aura around them while they are having intercourse. The atmosphere is practically identical to the purple timberland of fantasy trees with leaves and blossoms that structure a bend over the two accomplices. This makes incredible vibrations that consume with smoldering heat negative karmas. Mostly cherishing an individual and demonstrating this adoration through sex that is fulfilling can create anybody by and by and profoundly.

Reiki - The Energy Which Heals The Body

Two individuals put their hands directly over my body and following a few medicines during the day, I felt like another individual at night.

How is mending made? Individuals utilize the chakras of their hands to move vitality to the chakras of other individuals' body.

A chakra is a point of vitality situated in a particular position in our body. We have numerous purposes of energy (focuses where power comes in and goes out). Chinese medicine reports a lot over these focuses.

These focuses are a few, and vitality goes through them along vitality lines.

Among these, there are primary concerns that are called Chakras.

There are seven chakras in the body of every one of us. It is interesting, yet seven are the principal hues and melodic notes. Truth be told all known to man is represented by waves which are described by seven frequencies.

When we sing the seven melodic notes, we energize our chakras. This is the best strategy to use to distinguish our chakras.

Reiki has in the hundreds of years become a kind of medicine, and the individuals who are prepared can with the time become master in gathering vitality from the universe and moving it to different bodies. This is the fundamental guideline of Reiki: get energy and drive to others.

One can likewise get the vitality from the universe through his hands and move it to other possess chakras. You get the energy in the chakras of hands and run, for example to the chakra of the stomach. This procedure isn't anything but difficult to do. You need preparing, and a long haul works out.

There is likewise another critical perspective to consider. To be fruitful, Reiki needs that the healer and the individual to be mended are loose. The first segment of contemplation is suggested.

There are a few reasons why Reiki turned out to be so prevalent nowadays. Above all else, anybody can do Reiki accepting amends. It isn't expected to build up the capacity concerning different orders where the utilization of contemplation or different procedures are mentioned.

All Reiki procedures are passed on from instructors to understudies through an amends procedure beginning with the person who previously directed the method.

At long last there isn't have to drive the vitality, with Reiki the vitality streams suddenly guided and goes where required. Besides, on account of these qualities, Reiki ends up mainstream because can't incite agony or harms.

The individuals who do Reiki experience a non-intrusive type of mending and understand expansion in vitality in the body and mine and a superior condition of wellbeing. Their method for living is all the more unwinding.

The understudies begin their action with commencement to turn into a channel for the Reiki vitality. In the beginning, the activity is classified "expiation" and the novice experiences the same number of penances as they are essential to make the vitality move through his/her body. The subsequent stage for the understudy is to realize how to make Reiki medicines.

Brainwave Entrainment Can Unblock Your Crown Chakra

Brainwave entrainment is a neuro-innovative medium that modifies your brainwaves to mirror a particular recurrence, that will open and unblock your Crown Chakra, quickly and safely.

The Crown Chakra is a road to higher conditions of cognizance. Whenever open, it enables you to go to a spot past self-image, thought, feeling, and body, bringing more concordance and harmony into your life.

`Formative Age

The Crown is open in youthful youngsters the cover between our physical world and the astral domain is free for them.

It closes when a tyke is told, persistently, that what they see is only their creative mind.

It can start to grow once more, gradually, sparingly, at age 7 or 8.

This chakra can open again as an otherworldly grown-up, and be utterly dynamic by age 43 to 49.

Or, it might never open in specific individuals' lifetimes.

What Blocks a Crown Chakra?

The ailment is brought about by constant, over and again blocked chakra vitality.

Every one of the seven chakras holds the majority of your high and terrible musings, deeds, and activities that you have submitted in the majority of your lifetimes.

Suppression of feelings causes torment, enduring and sickness, and the hindering of the crown chakra.

A few explanations behind a blocked Crown Chakra.

Memories, possibly not by any means conscious recollections, of youth injury.

Any injury as a kid will reflect issues of pardoning and feeling acknowledged.

Abuse.

Learned prohibitive conviction frameworks.

Emotional injury as a tyke will happen as blocked feelings sometime down the road.

If you experience difficulty tolerating yourself, odds are you were dismissed as a tyke.

Many of your feelings of dread started at the ages of 7 or 8, and if you confronted last analysis, your Crown would wind up hindered.

Emotional wounds that haven't been pardoned.

Lack of consideration.

If pressure develops at one of the lower six chakras, from rehashed blame, disavowal, restraint, or unfelt feelings, the Crown is influenced.

If there is a division from your dad, the Crown closes, and you feel a feeling of disconnection and aloneness, that just can't be smothered.

How a Blocked Crown Chakra Manifests Into The Physical

A blocked Crown obstructs the progression of Divine light to move through the body, influencing stance, digestion, breathing, and your enthusiastic state.

A shiver, throb, or affectability in any of the districts administered by the Crown, (pineal organ, cerebral cortex, focal sensory system, right eye, all pieces of the cerebrum, pituitary organ, hair development), is brought about by uncertain feelings put away around there. When the serious subject matter has been settled, the pulse will vanish. The quality of the hurt is legitimately corresponding to the size of the issue.

Butterflies-feeling as if something is moving within you, or attempting to.

Intense or dull weight, cerebral pain, or headache, beginning at the Crown.

If you experience the ill effects of headaches, you experience difficulty living at the time, the mantra of an open Crown Chakra.

Can trigger discouragement, disarray, feebleness, the dread of achievement, absence of motivation, intellectualizing, and profound compulsion.

Chakra Opening With Crystals and Brainwave Entrainment

In the modern world, we will see in general disregard our vitality frameworks, which frequently turned out to be over-burden and focused, and therefore we become exhausted and begin to fail to meet expectations in our work.

The body's vitality framework is upheld by an arrangement of hubs which are known as the chakras, and it is the point at which they become obstructed that you will feel sick. By unblocking and opening up your chakras, you will feel re-stimulated and ready to last during that time without your vitality getting to be drained. With the present hectic ways of life, this could easily compare to ever. Working on your chakras can likewise build up your dormant clairvoyant vitality.

There are seven principle chakra focuses, which you can take a shot at and they are related with specific hues:

1. The base chakra is arranged at the base of the spine and is related to red and for adjusting physical vitality. This chakra will likewise ground you and help with inspiration.

2. The sacral chakra is arranged in the lower abdomen beneath the navel and is related with the shading orange. This is to discharge squares and create innovativeness.

3. The sun-powered plexus chakra is arranged around the lower ribcage and is related with the shading yellow. Taking a shot at this chakra will create certainty and true discernment.

4. The heart chakra is related to shading green. The heart chakra will build up a feeling of direction throughout everyday life and improve associations with others.

5. The throat chakra is related to the shading blue. This chakra is associated with correspondence and tranquility and how you convey what needs be to the world.

6. The temples chakra amidst the brow is related to the shading indigo. This is the chakra related to mental and natural exercises and chipping away at this chakra will encourage the opening of the third eye.

7. The crown chakra is related to purple. This is the chakra identified with the entire being and equalizations the majority of the faculties of self, profound, physical, passionate, and mental. Taking a shot at this chakra will build up an association

with your higher self and lead to a higher scholarly association.

Each of these chakras is vortices of vitality, which can be invigorated by utilizing gems and mental perception.

Precious stones can be utilized to open up chakras by resting comfortably on the floor and putting a gem related with the shade of each of the chakras on the suitable position of the body. Inhale gradually and unwind while picturing the shading associated with each chakra.

There are different guided chakra purifying activities and contents which can be utilized for chakra opening, yet the ideal approach to check out the vitality examples is to consolidate the chakra working with brainwave entrainment. Working with your chakras along these lines will give your entire body a revitalizing jolt of energy and make you all the more rationally alert just as honing your intuitive faculties.

Chapter 2: The Current State Of Reiki Training

At present and in the West, the training given to Reiki students has lost much of its content, trivializing, mitigating and mimicking other techniques. We cannot deny that the wide and rapid expansion of this technique in addition to carrying these undesirable consequences will have contributed in some way to enrich and mature the technique. Despite this, it would be desirable to recover the contents that in many cases have been neglected or, directly, are unknown.

Currently, a typical first-grade Reiki seminar takes place in about sixteen hours that are spread over a weekend. The theoretical contents are limited to teaching some version of the history of Reiki, the Principles of Reiki and the positions of the hands to perform the treatments. The practical part usually consists of the exchange of treatments between the assistants to the course and the accomplishment of works of visualization, relaxation or meditation with the purpose of infusing in the assistants a mood favorable to the reception of the initiation. In some cases, participants in the course are offered the possibility of continuing to practice for a period after the end of the course. Contents of an ethical or philosophical type are non-existent or are stained by the commercial ideas mentioned at the beginning of these letters and leave aside the formality that a subject like the one being treated deserves: the health (balance) of the person.

I do not intend to judge these seminars, because thanks to them, many people are receiving a tool of great value for themselves and their close people, but if we stop to compare the goal of initiation to the first level of Reiki (the harmonization of the person) with the means offered in these seminars, we have no choice but to recognize that the latter is not sufficient to achieve the goal set.

Reiki is a simple system, which does not require a great knowledge to be applied. As it is usually said in the literature on the subject: no special qualities are necessary for its practice and anyone can do it. In the usual seminar of a weekend, it is possible to acquire the technical knowledge about the application of Reiki and, through the process of initiations, the ability to channel Reiki. But is this enough? Is this limited to what a person who will take responsibility for their own health should receive? Do we stop to think that, over time, this person will not only treat himself and his family but can start giving Reiki to other people?

We can limit the Reiki seminar to the transmission of basic technical knowledge and the ability to channel, but then we have to be honest with the people who attend and inform them, at least, that it is not enough to undergo daily self-treatment with Reiki to maintain optimal health in all aspects.

There are many people who attend Reiki seminars with a background of previous knowledge and are already able to take care of themselves properly. But we must not forget that there are many people for whom Reiki, for different reasons, is the first contact with their responsibility for their own health. Many people who had never needed information about how to feed themselves or how to take care of their attitude in everyday activities. These people arrive at the Reiki seminar without a clear awareness of the influence that these and other issues have on their state of health and, unfortunately, it is not difficult for them to finish the seminar in the same state. We must recognize that this same circumstance occurs in courses and seminars of other therapies, but it is from Reiki what we are dealing with at the moment.

In these circumstances, many newcomers often go through difficult or discouraging experiences: they practice Reiki regularly but the improvements are not too consistent or make themselves wait, they go through phases of apparent or real deterioration that cannot understand or confuse physical sensations outside Reiki with consequences of it. This is compounded by the fact that there has not been time for a healthy personal bond to be created between the Reiki teacher and his apprentice, it is normal for his contacts to be reduced to the few hours of the seminars; so the newcomer tries to clarify his doubts in the literature on the subject, full of contradictions and influences of other techniques and possibly only increase the disorientation of the new practitioner.

It is not uncommon for a person who is in these circumstances to abandon the practice of Reiki because of discontent or distrust, which can only be considered a failure attributable to the corresponding teacher. Thus, it would be desirable for Reiki seminars, specifically those of first level training, to offer a more complete preparation and according to what one would expect, without ceasing to be accessible to the large and heterogeneous public that shows interest in them.

Chapter 3: The Root Chakra

To be connected to the Root Chakra, you must connect with your physical endurance, vitality, and mental perseverance. The Root Chakra is the center of your passion and connects directly to your existence. If you want to align your Root Chakra, you must evaluate your life to determine if you're physically fit, have been or are currently being abused verbally or physically, are able to act on your thoughts, are able to accomplish your goals, place importance on your home and money, and have thought of self-destruction recently.

To boost the Root Chakra power and encourage the flow of Red energy, you must include physical activities like yoga or exercise in your daily or weekly regimen. You must eat and drink red food and drinks. You can use aromatherapy oils like juniper, ylang ylang, or sandalwood. Latin American music and drumbeats can stimulate the Root Chakra. Red stones like ruby, red jasper, garnet, or red tiger's eye can be worn or carried. Furthermore, you can use red in your artworks, décor, color bath, and clothes.

The Root Chakra is closely associated with the color red. Its Sanskrit name is Muladhara and is located at the base of the spine. It is responsible for your survival instinct and deals with tasks connected to the physical and material world. It empowers you to stand up for yourself. It also pertains to security issues. An imbalanced Root Chakra can manifest itself through depression, sciatica, lower back pain, fatigue, anemia, cold feet, cold hand, and frequent colds.

The Root Chakra is also known as the security center. Its exact location in the body is the perineum, which is that part between the sex organ and the anus. Other parts of the body which are connected to this chakra center are the lower extremities, the bladder and elimination system, the sacral plexus, the skeleton system, the lymph system, and the men's prostate gland. Also, the nose is part of the Root Chakra because it is connected with survival and it is for your sense of smell. The adrenal glands are also part of this chakra center.

The Root Chakra is connected to that part of your consciousness pertaining to job, home, money, trust, survival, and security. If it is balanced, you will be grounded, present in the here and now, and can feel secure. If the chakra is tensed, you can experience fear or feel insecure. You may feel threatened if this tension becomes worse. If there are symptoms in the elimination system, the legs, and the skeletal system, there may be tensions in this chakra center. This means that you are living in fear or insecurity. If one leg isn't functioning properly or it is feeling pained, you may have trust issues. It is easy to find out what is causing the leg problems because the symptoms develop at the time of the happening of an event or circumstance. Furthermore, if the sense of smell is affected, it also means that there are tensions in the Root Chakra.

The Earth is its associated element. The Root Chakra reflects how you associate with the Earth. It is also connected with how you relate to your mother. If you are separated from your mother or if you feel unloved by your mother, the Root Chakra can be tensed. The tension will be eased if you feel loved by your mother again.

The Root Chakra is responsible for your physical awareness and your feeling of comfort in various situations. If this chakra is opened, you will feel secure, stable, sensible, and well-balanced. You will trust people around you. You will feel present in the now and physically connected to your body. If the chakra is overactive, you may feel greedy, materialistic and may not welcome change. The body can be used to open the Root Chakra. You can do some manual housecleaning, walk around the block or do some yoga exercises. These activities will strengthen the chakra and let you become one with your own body once again.

Grounding is also a good way of opening the chakra. This means that you must feel the earth beneath you. You must be able to connect with the ground. To become grounded you must first stand relaxed and straight. The feet must be apart and the distance between them must be equal to shoulder width. Next, you must bend your knees slightly. The pelvis must be moved forward while keeping the body balanced. The weight must be evenly distributed through the feet. Next sink your weight forward while maintaining the position for a few minutes.

Afterwards, you can sit cross-legged, the tips of the index finger and thumb must tough gently. You must concentrate on your Root Chakra and its meaning. You then chant "LAM" in a clear yet silent manner. Let yourself relax while thinking about the chakra until you feel completely relaxed. Next, you must visualize a red flower, which is closed. You must imagine that there is a powerful energy coming from it and that its four petals are slightly opening with full energy. The perineum must be contracted while holding your breath then slowly releasing it.

Chapter 4: The Three Pillars Of Reiki

Dr. Usui taught us three pillars of Reiki: Gassho, Reiji-Ho, and Chiryo. These three pillars are used as the foundation of your Reiki practice.

Gassho

The first pillar of Reiki is Gassho.

Gassho means two hands coming together. It is the prayer position, with your palms together in the steeple position, in front of your chest. It is wonderful to think about the many cultures around the world (and throughout time) that have used the prayer position to give thanks, gratitude, and respect, and to bring focus. In Gassho, you use this position to connect to Reiki and the universal ki.

Dr. Usui recommended that the Gassho meditation be done daily in the morning (before starting your day) and in the evening (at the close of your day) for 15-30 minutes. In Chapter 7, there are a number of guided Reiki meditations you can use for healing, centering, and wellness - including a daily Gassho meditation. You also use Gassho for a few short moments at the beginning of each Reiki healing session. This practice focuses your intent and invites in the Reiki healing energy.

To Practice Gassho At The Beginning Of A Reiki Treatment

At the beginning of the session, take a moment to close your eyes.

Bring your hands together, upright, at chest level.

Focus your attention on the tips of your third fingers (or between your palms).

Breathe in the Reiki energy and feel it filling the space between your palms.

Exhale and feel the Reiki flowing into your body – your physical and energy body.

Calm and centered, continue to breathe in the Reiki energy and feel it flowing through you.

Keep your focus on your third fingers.

Set your intention for the session.

After a few moments, open your eyes.

Reiji-Ho

The second pillar of Reiki is Reiji-Ho.

Reiji means the indication of the Reiki energy. Ho means process. Reiji-Ho is the guidance of the Reiki energy during treatment. In this pillar of Reiki, you let go of your ego and your own pre-conceived notions of what needs to be treated and let the Reiki guide you.

To Practice Reiji-Ho:

After completing Gassho, lift your hands in prayer position to your forehead and silently ask for Reiki to guide the session and for healing to occur in the person you are treating.

The Reiki will guide you to where treatment is needed. Let go. Let go of your ego, let go of your thoughts. You are the hollow reed that Reiki flows through.

Reiki will flow and draw you to where it is needed. This may feel like a gentle nudging, a magnet drawing you, or a subtle intuition. In the beginning, you will use the prescribed positions for treatment, however as you grow in your practice, you will rely more on Reiji-Ho. You may continue to always treat all the positions, or you may add or remove depending on how Reiji-Ho guides you.

This practice, of following the guidance of Reiki, is Reiji-Ho.

Chiryo

Chiryo means treatment. This is the step in which you allow Reiki to flow freely through you and give healing energy to you (in self-treatment) or to the recipient. Chiryo is the actual treatment or delivery of Reiki during a session.

As you move through the treatment positions, Reiki will flow freely and strongly in areas where it is needed. When the Reiki tapers off, you can move to the next position. After all the positions have been treated sufficiently you will be guided to end the treatment.

You may also choose to utilize a specific type of Chiryo for detoxification. This involves removing energetic, emotional or physical "toxins" from the body. These toxins can be mental blocks, emotional blocks or trauma, physical symptoms and pain, or any other "toxin" needing to be cleared from the body.

To Practice Detoxifying Chiryo

Place your right hand above the crown chakra (top of the head) and your left hand above the tanden (slightly below the navel on the abdomen). Set the intention that all "toxins" be cleared from the body. Leave your hands in this position until you feel a balance and a free flow of energy between your hands.

Chapter 7 includes a meditation that can assist in clearing toxins from the body during a Chiryo detoxification.

Once you have completed Chiryo/Reiki treatment, close with a short Gassho meditation of gratitude for the healing.

Finish with an energetic cleansing of you and the recipient.

Aura Cleansing

Once you have finished the Reiki treatment you can clear your aura of any stagnant energies that were released during the treatment.

To Cleanse Your Energy And Remove Stagnant Energies

Take your right hand and wipe across your chest from the upper right chest to the lower left abdomen.

Take your left hand and wipe across your chest from the upper left chest to the lower right abdomen.

Next, take your right hand and sweep down from the left shoulder to the left palm.

Then, take your left hand and sweep down from the right shoulder to the right palm.

Finally, shake out your hands, like you are flinging away drops of water.

Go and wash your hands with soap and water. You have combed out your aura and freed it of stagnant energies.

To Cleanse The Energy And Remove Stagnant Energies In Another

Sweep your fingers (one to four inches above the body) from the head down to the left arm, then from the head down the right arm.

Comb down the chest.

Sweep your hands from the abdomen down the left leg, then from the abdomen down the right leg.

Sweep your fingers down the entire energy field.

Repeat as many times as feels necessary.

Shake out your hands as if you are flinging away drops of water.

You have combed the aura and freed it of stagnant energies.

Key Take Away

Reiki treatment is composed of three pillars: Gassho, Reiji-Ho and Chiryo. Gassho is a meditation and focused intent that invites Reiki to begin healing. Reiji-Ho is following the guidance of Reiki during treatment. Chiryo is the actual treatment. These three pillars make up the Reiki session.

Chapter 5: Body Energy Systems

For all it's imperfections, the physical body and it's connection to being has evolved into something quite astounding. A near perfect combination of energy structures working together in harmony to create every amazing part and ability of your body.

When the energy structures are working together as they should, everything about the body is good. The body is in good health and performing at peak efficiency. When the energy structures are not, things tend to not function as well. The body will get sick, experience pain and when the structures break down enough, the body will die.

Because these structures are interconnected, they are able to coordinate in an intelligent fashion. This occurs because energy pathways running throughout the entire body, enables multidirectional interactive communication. Something that happens on one side of the body is communicated throughout the body near instantaneously. This is why it is possible for you to treat a headache by ingesting a pain killer through your mouth. Seemingly disconnected, yet connected because it is connected to the entire body.

When treating a body with Reiki it works the same. You provide healing energy and the body applies that energy where needed, restoring and correcting connections in the life force along the way.

In the same way as the pain killer distributes itself through the body, so does the healing energy provided. Unlike the painkiller however, the energy can be provided in direct physical proximity to the area affected, reducing the dilution affect resulting from distance between source and destination. The healing energy available is also not finite like a pain killer.

Life Force Defaults

At any given moment in time, your life force has a base default energy position. This is the position at which your energy structures are as near to perfect harmony as your connection between soul and body will permit. Whatever energy position your body finds itself in at any given moment, it will always attempt to reset to this default. It may not always be able to do so without help, but it will try.

Living within the constraints of a physical body however means a constant onslaught on your energy system harmony. Every breath that you take, every meal that you eat and every step you take, impacts this.

When you eat something unhealthy, it moves your body away from harmony. When you get sick, this occurred due to disharmony. Pain is an identifiable symptom of disharmony.

The harmony points are ever changing. As you grow and evolve your harmony points grow and evolve with you. Harmony points are affected by several factors including genetics, life experiences and other external impacts over time.

When treating a body with Reiki, the healing energy provided will be used by the body to help it restore itself to those default harmony points. The inherent body intelligence ensures that the healing energy will be used where it is needed.

Working with Energy

A simple thought. Like a seed growing from your mind, flowing through your body, directed where you want it to go. This is the act of Reiki.

Without another Reiki practitioner to assist you with learning this skill, you may find this a little challenging. Once you become familiar with the physical sensations that stem from the act of manipulating energy however, it is easily repeated.

If you are alone, place your hands in a prayer position in front of your body (heart center position).

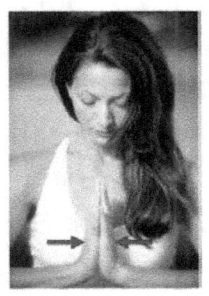

When thinking about moving energy, think of it as if it is water flowing from your arms through into the palms of your hands. Avoid physically increasing the pressure of your hands. Just hold them lightly together.

From both sides (with your thoughts) open the flow and direct energy towards the palms of your hands. Let the energy connect where your palms connect. See it. Feel it.

You should notice after a bit that the palms of your hands are starting to feel warmer than they should naturally from just holding them together. The more energy you direct towards your hands, the more heat will be generated. You should also start to notice a slight prickly / tingly sensation in both your palms and likely some of the fingers. If you do, you have just recognized for the first time what it feels like to direct energy.

When you start to recognize these sensations, using Reiki becomes much easier. After just a little practice, you will notice that to get energy moving, all you have to do is think it so.

Energy can also be transmitted directionally. To enhance your ability to sense energy flows, holding the same hand positions, direct the energy to flow to one side and then the other repeatedly. Doing so will feel different and the sensation of receiving versus pushing should become easily distinguishable.

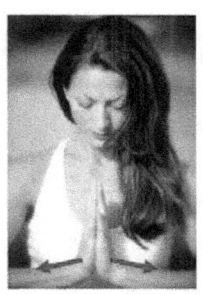

Not unlike anything else, the more you practice, the better you will get at recognizing energy movement. The better you get at recognizing it's movement, the better you will get at transmitting it.

You will also start to notice that the Reiki sensations in your hands happen, even if your hands are not in the prayer (heart center) position. Just think about it to make it happen. Trust yourself and your ability to recognize it.

Another more visual symptom of moving energy through your hands is that the skin on your palms will become slightly spotty and when you start moving larger quantities of energy, your palms might actually feel itchy. Shake it off just like water.

With practice you can turn it on and off at will. It is controlled by your thoughts. Think it so and it will be.

Reiki can be projected from anywhere in your body, though projection from the palms of your hands will feel natural and be fairly easy to master. Focus your efforts on learning how to do this first.

Chapter 6: Basic Yoga Postures

Pre Position

Standing position

Sitting position

Supine position

Prone position (lying straight head bent down)

Asana for beginners

Hasta Sanchalan (movement of arms)

Type 1: Take shavanasana pose (corpse pose), keep hand away at a distance of 6-7 inches with leg separated apart to 12 inches. Now lift the hand from the ground and take it towards your head, keep the forearms crossed and hands parallel to ground. Now raise the arms above up in air and then slowly bring them on stomach and then to normal position.

Type2: Take shavanasana pose (corpse pose), keep hand away at a distance of 6-7 inches and leg separated apart to 12 inches. Now lift the hand from ground and take them up towards head. Now stretch hands upwards and leg downwards for about 5 sec. Then slowly without and jerk bring back hands to normal position. Repeat this in the same manner.

This movement helps in strengthening the neck, back and shoulders.
Pada Sanchalan (movement of legs)

Type 1: Take supine position. Keeping hands close to your body, without bending the knee lift right leg up to an angle of 30 degree, then bring it to normal position. Do the same exercise with left leg.

Type 2: Take supine position, take your hands at the same level of shoulders (both should be at same height, parallel to the ground). Lift your left leg and stretch it towards right side as much as possible without bending the knees and touch the ground. Do the same exercise with right leg.

This movement helps the development of knee muscles and knee joints.

Janu Sanchalan (movement of knees)

Type 1: Take supine position; slowly move hands around the head. Slowly bend your left leg knee in a way that the foot is placed near hip. Now move the knee to opposite direction, i.e. to right side as much as possible. Do the same with right leg.

Type 2: Take supine position; slowly move hands around the head. Slowly bend both legs knee one by one in a way that the foot is placed near hip. Now stretch towards the left side of your body in a way that the left knee touches the ground.

Repeat the same action in the opposite direction. Keep repeating 4-5 times. Slowly bring the hands to normal.

These movements' benefits knee joints, spine and hip joints to relax.

Skandha Sanchalan (movement of shoulders)

Type 1: Take vajrasana position. Keeping the body straight, put your arms by the side and then, without jerking, lift both the shoulders up towards your ears, and then bring it slowly to normal position.

Type 2: Take vajrasana position. Keeping your body straight, keep your left hand on left shoulder by making a fist and right hand on right shoulder. Bring the elbows together to chest. Now slowly start rotating both the arms in opposite directions (one in clockwise and another in anti-clockwise). Now repeat it in opposite direction.

This movement is helpful for people with back problem.

Datta Mudra (movement of neck)

Sit down in vajrasana position with hands on the knees and head straight in same line. Turn your neck to left stretching as much as possible. Then come back to now position slowly bringing head straight. Now turn to right side stretching maximum. Return to normal position.

Brahma Mudra (movement of neck)

It depicts the three gods of creation, protection and destruction through our asana. Sit clasping the leg one on one another with hands straight on knee and look straight. Now slowly turn your head towards right direction. Then bring it back straight and then turn towards left finally bringing them straight.

Kantha Sanchalan (movement of neck)

Type 1: Take Vajrasana position (kneeling pose), keeping neck straight first bend forward without jerking yourself, then take to the normal position. In the same way bend left then go back to normal position, then slowly to right side. **Type 2:** Take Vajrasana position, keeping neck straight without jerking yourself start rotating the neck clockwise from left side then taking it backside and then to right slowly bringing it to front. Again repeat it in anticlockwise direction from right side of shoulder.

Caution: This should not be tried by people suffering from spondylitis.

Shavasana (corpse pose)

Lie straight on your back with legs apart with a distance of 1-1.5 inches with fingers pointed opposite direction. Keep your hand raised in line to your shoulder with palms facing upwards. Now Inhale and hold your breath for a while. Try taking the inhaled air to your cheeks by pressing lips, tightening abdomen, tensing your ears and wrinkled forehead.

Exhale and calm yourself so that the tension from your body is absorbed by the floor. Get back to normal position.

Swastikasana (auspicious pose)

This is the most important and easiest asana for meditation. Sit with leg crossed and with feet between the thighs, and hands on the knees, straight in chin mudra. This helps in giving relaxation to people with varicose vein problem.

Sukha Pranayam (deep breathing)

Sit in swastikasana (meditation pose). It is about observing your breath to feel the energy. Breathe normally and observe the atmosphere. Concentrate on your breathing and abdominal movement. Slowly make sure when your inhale the abdominal wall moves out and while exhaling it moves in. Here imagine when you inhale all the energy goes in and while exhaling it is all the stress, disease going out.

Tadagasana (pond pose)

Take supine position and bring the heels close to hip by bending the knee. Keep hands around the head. Take normal breath. Now come back to original position.

Vajrasana (thunderbolt pose)

Sit on heels with knee pointed straight and calves under the thigh. The toes of leg should touch each other and the hands should be on the knee cap with distance between the fingers. This asana is used for various meditation processes.

Janu Hastasana (hand to knee pose)

Sit in vajrasana position and place both the palms on the ground in front of knees next to each other. Now breathe normally by pushing your head backward and chest forward and waist downward.

Adhavasana (Downward facing pose)

Stand straight with hands by your side. Now bend on your waist bringing hands forward and pressing the ground with fingers little apart from each other. Now look down and push your hips upwards making it an inverted V position.

Makaraasana (Crocodile pose)

Lie upside down, with legs apart to 1-1.5 inches with toes pointing upward and hand bended upward towards the head in a way that the head is rested on arms. Breathe normally.

Shishu asana (Child pose)

Sit on your heels and slowly bring your torso forward and make the head rest on the ground with hands in front of you parallel to each other. Now press your chest on your knees by lowering it. Hold for a while and relax to normal position.

Parvataasana (Mountain pose)

Stand straight keeping feet together and arms by the side. Distribute the body weight throughout your body. Now relax and slowly raise your hands upwards. Touch the sky with finger tips. Keep your arms straight with the palms facing each other.

Vriskshasana (Tree pose)

Stand straight with hands by your side. Now slowly keep the left leg foot on the right legs thigh (inner side of thigh) with hips facing forward. Then bring hand to your chest with palms together (prayer position). Now inhale and take arms upwards, slowly making the palms separate. Come to normal position and repeat the same action on another leg.

Trikonasana (Triangle pose)

Stand straight with hands in line of your shoulders extended sideways. Stand apart with about 2-3 inches gap between the legs. Slowly bend sideways making the right palm rest on the tight foot and left hand up in air straight and watch the ceiling. Hold the pose for a while and return back to normal position.

Sukhasana (Seated twist)

Sit on the floor and extend the left leg. Slowly, cross twist your right leg and keep the right foot behind left leg thigh with left knee bent touching right leg thigh. Let the toe of right leg be straight and upward. Now keep right hand on the floor by stretching sideways and left hand on the right thigh in a way the elbow touches the knee. Now stretch and twist your body right as much as u can without hurting yourself. Hold for a minute, breathe normally, and then come back to normal position. Do the same action with left side.

Chapter 7: The Reiki Attunements.

The very essence of a First Degree Reiki workshop is the four attunements (also known as initiations) that you will receive. During these, your physical and etheric bodies will be fine tuned to open up and your energy system, (also known as the chakras) will be aligned, to receive and channel Reiki, the Universal Life Force, by the application of an ancient method as taught by Dr. Usui.

When you receive your first attunement, energy will start flowing through your hands at the thought of healing. The last attunement will seal this empowerment in so your channels will stay open for the rest of your life. Once attuned the ability to heal is not lost, even if it is not used for years.

During the Second Degree you will receive a further two attunements. The reason for these attunements we will go into at a later date.

During your Master's Degree a further attunement is given.

There is not enough space within a small volume such as this to go into the details of the attunements, nor is it the right place.

These are the only attunements necessary in the practice of Reiki.

The Three Degrees of Reiki.

Reiki, as it is taught today, is divided into three parts or degrees: First Degree, Second Degree and the Master's Degree. Although it is necessary for everybody to start with First Degree Reiki, it is not necessary to do the other two degrees. First Degree Reiki is a complete system by itself and is often all that is needed. Unfortunately in our society there seems to be a desire to acquire qualifications and certificates even if we don't need them. It is rather like my computer or my video recorder. I only use a small part of their capabilities; the rest is a waste and an expensive one at that.

In searching for a way to explain how the degrees of traditional Reiki fit into our lives I have come up with the following analogy. Like all analogies it is not exactly right but gives an idea of how to view the degrees.

Imagine that you were born in a small village. If you are completely happy with yourself within the limits of that village, there is no need for change. But usually a time comes when you want to travel and go a little beyond the distance that is sensible to walk. So you decide to learn to drive and buy a car. First you must learn to drive. This represents the time you join a First Degree Reiki workshop. Here you are shown how the car works and how to use it on the road. Passing your test and buying a little car represents completion of your First Degree.

With more than a little trepidation you go for your first drive. It may be just around the block and you find that it is different to sitting in a dual controlled car with an instructor. Now it is all down to you. Sensibly you stick closely to what you have learnt because it works and it gives you confidence.

Driving alone in the car is when you really start to understand what driving is all about. Sometimes your ego steps in and you try to do something your way. Sometimes this is fine and it works, other times you make a real pig's ear of it. It's all part of the learning process, gaining experience and confidence and trusting yourself in all situations of driving until it becomes second nature and comfortable and you can sit back and enjoy the trip.

You make friends with your little car and it gets you around the village just fine. It can take you on further journeys to other places. In fact your car can take you where ever you wish to go. Being a small car it may take time and it has its' limitations.

Time changes and you decide to take up a musical instrument; a double bass. Now fitting a double bass into a very small car is an interesting problem. What's more you have to travel all over the place to attend concerts and go to teachers, etc. You need a different type of car to do this sort of work. So you buy a Volvo Estate. The Volvo still does all the work that your other little car did but now you can also easily travel with your double bass up to Scotland and back. It can move more and go faster. It costs more to run so unless you need it it's better to stay with your small car.

After a while you find that you really like driving and would like to make a career of it. Maybe become a driving instructor and teach others to drive. To do this takes quite a bit of commitment; you must really want to teach others before you start, as it involves quite an outlay in terms of time, money and commitment. With a bit of luck the moment of madness passes and you go back to playing your double base and enjoying life. If it doesn't and you become a driving instructor you need yet another car. It has to do all the jobs your car did before but now it has to have dual controls so that you can teach others to drive safely. All these stages involve driving but each stage needs a different vehicle and a different approach. They are all based upon that initial driving test, this is a must. But unless you need the space to carry a double base or intend to teach others to drive you can stay with a simpler vehicle. It is not necessary to be a driving instructor to enjoy driving, or to drive well.

The Reiki Degrees just allow you to do different things. While they are all complete units they all evolve out of the First Degree. What you do after that is up to you.

It is not necessary to hold all three degrees in Reiki. It is not a ladder that must be climbed in order to gain proficiency. There are many people with First Degree Reiki who are more confident and more efficient users of Reiki than some Masters. They use that part of the Reiki training which is relevant and have gained a greater understanding and wisdom of Reiki because of this focus.

Chapter 8: Symbols And Attunements

WHAT ARE SYMBOLS?

Reiki symbols are sacred healing symbols that enhance the flow of life force energy. They are like keys that open doors to higher levels of awareness and manifestation. After Reiki Level 2 training, practitioners learn how to use specific symbols **to guide and focus the transfer of energy.**

Reiki symbols are Sanskrit-derived Japanese forms. Sanskrit is the mother tongue of all other languages. It is the language of the Vedas, which are some of the oldest writings known to man. The Vedas say Sanskrit is the language of the spirit world.

Reiki symbols are shown to the student prior to being attuned. An imprinting takes place that links the image they are shown to the metaphysical energies the symbol represents. Then, the Reiki attunement actually empowers the symbols so they fulfill their intended purpose. This process has been created by a Divine covenant, or sacred agreement, between the Creator and those who have been attuned.

WHAT ARE ATTUNEMENTS?

We are born with the potential to channel life force energy, but most require the attunement process offered by a Reiki Master Teacher to be realigned with the energy. This is achieved by a number of attunements during which the individual's own energy field and chakra system is literally tuned in to receive the waves of Universal Life Energy in much the same way that you would tune in a radio station to receive another frequency. Once attuned, the flow of energy is turned on simply by placing the hands on oneself or on someone else. Touch is the signal for switching the energy on. Being attuned to Reiki makes the energy readily available to the channel during their life.

You become empowered. You can receive and channel larger doses of energy.

REIKI BLESSINGS

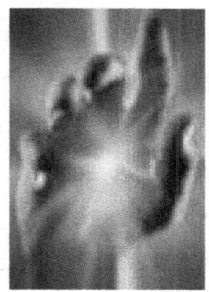

Reiju: Attunements are Reiki blessings, a form of empowerment, passed on regularly from teacher to student that help the student move through any areas of resistance that may prevent a student from deepening his or her practice. The teacher, through regular practice, becomes a facilitator to help move stagnant energy within the student. This occurs on a periodic basis throughout a student's training until becoming a Reiki Master. At this point, the student will have all the tools, awareness and energetic control to be of service to their own students.

Often times , **attunements are considered a ceremonial rite of passage** for the Reiki student. The teacher symbolically passes along an energetic awareness by freeing up any constrictions and dense energies. Tools are also provided for the student to utilize in healing one's self and others.

Attunements are necessary to elevate the student to the next level of their personal and professional practice.
FOUR EMPOWERING ATTUNEMENTS

In Reiki Level 1, you receive four attunements over the course of two days minimum. This is to balance and fine tune your physical body, raising the vibrational level at the cellular structure. This enables you to receive and channel larger dosages of energy. The endocrine system is positively affected. Benefits continue due to toxins leaving during the 21-day cleansing process. Your Reiki channel as a giver and receiver are with you for life. If you do not regularly practice, it may become like a stiff muscle until you loosen it up with a renewed connection and practice.

Dr. Laxmi Horan states in **Exploring Reiki**:

"The purpose of the attunements is not to open chakras or awaken the Kundalini, although sometimes certain openings may occur. The focus of First Degree attunements is to reinstate the Reiki channel, the direct link we've always had (but could not perceive due to our conditioning) to the Universal Life Force Energy which we truly are."

Below is a further summary from **Exploring Reiki** regarding the empowerment process. You will receive the following four attunements during your Level 1 training.

The First Attunement

 The heart and the thymus on the physical and etheric levels are affected.

The Second Attunement

On the physical level, the thyroid and parathyroid glands become attuned. On the etheric level, the communication and truth centers are open. The nervous system also receives a boost of energy and undergoes an adjustment period.

The Third Attunement

The effects are felt at the pineal gland located at the third eye point and hypothalamus, which is responsible for the body's moods and regulating the body's temperature. Many initiates experience visions and see colors and symbols. An overwhelming sense of serenity is experienced.

The Fourth Attunement

The final empowerment seals in and encapsulates all the higher energies that your system has accepted. It has completely become part of your totality. You are now deeply connected to Reiki.

Japanese Cleansing

The following techniques were taught by Dr. Usui to all his students. The following text is a combination from William Rand, founder of The International Centre for Reiki Training, and **The Japanese Art of Reiki** by Bronwen and Frans Stiene.

THE KENYOKU HO: DRY BATHING METHOD

This technique cleanses yourself of any negative energy you have picked up from anyone, or simply to cleanse your field of constricted energy patterns. It strengthens your energy while completely cleansing you. It is good to do kenyoku before beginning treatment and at the end to disconnect from the client's energy. It can be practiced on its own or as a precursor to another energetic practice.

To begin:
1. Sit or stand.
2. Fix your eyes on the floor.
3. Release tension from the body.
4. Bring the mental focus to the hara (navel center).
5. Allow the hands to rise to gassho (prayer pose). There are two parts to this technique.

Part I

1. Place your right hand on the left shoulder (where the collarbone and shoulder meet).

2. Breathe in, and while exhaling, slowly and deliberately sweep your right hand diagonally down and across the torso to the right hip and off the body. In this large sweep, the energy from the left shoulder, heart, stomach and liver is cleared. Leave your right hand on your right hip.

3. Do the same with the left hand moving up to the right shoulder and stroking down to the left hip. Now the energy from the right shoulder, heart, stomach and spleen has been cleared.
 YOU MAY REPEAT SEVERAL TIMES.

Part II

1. Place your bent left elbow against your side with your forearm straight out in

front, horizontal to the ground. Your left palm is flat, facing upward and level to the ground as if you are balancing a plate on it.

2. Place your right hand at top of the left arm.

3. Breathe in, and while exhaling, sweep downward along the arm through the crook of the elbow, across the palm to the fingertips, and off the hands.

4. Repeat this action with the other side of the body.
5. To finish, bring your hands into gassho (prayer pose).

Every emotion and belief runs through the chakra and is distributed to our cells, tissues, and organs.

Overview oftheChakras

Your body contains seven main energy centers known as **chakras.** Though there are many, many more, these seven represent the general state of our being.

The word chakra is derived from Sanskrit, meaning wheel. This is because chakras are spinning vortexes of energy. They are located within our **etheric body**. It is through the etheric body that we receive, transmit and process life energies—similar to doorways through which we manifest emotional, mental and spiritual forces into physical expression. Every emotion and belief runs through the chakra and is distributed to our cells, tissues, and organs. Each chakra relates to physical, emotional, mental, and spiritual energies, as well as specific aspects of our consciousness.

The chakras are associated with the endocrine glands and the seven colors of the rainbow spectrum. Understanding the chakras helps to integrate all aspects of our consciousness that create a complete unit— the physical, material, sexual, mental and spiritual.

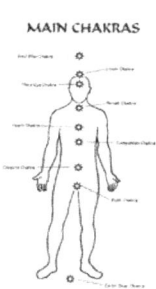

EARTH STAR CHAKRA

Located just below earth level and between your feet. Connects you to Mother Earth and allows you to flow with Her natural rhythms.

FIRST CHAKRA: ROOT

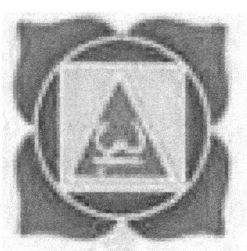

The root chakra is the system's foundation. We are involved with our survival and safety: having and possessing. We project and manifest our worldly needs through our ability to ground energy within our body.

Location The perineum – at the base of the spine
Color Red
Element Earth
Functions Basic needs, stability, security, survival, instincts, emotions (fear, calm)
Glands Adrenals
Body Parts Kidneys, spinal column, colon, large intestine, legs, bones, immune

system

Gems/Mineral Ruby, garnet, bloodstone, red jasper, black tourmaline, obsidian, smoky quartz

Foods Proteins, red fruits and vegetables

When Balanced

Good health, body confidence, no financial worries, easy flow of money, all needs are met, ability to trust in a Higher Power

When Imbalanced

Compromised health (especially lower back and sciatica), weight issues, poor diet, financial debt, ungrounded, detached from nature

SECOND CHAKRA: CREATIVE

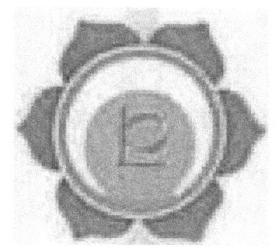

Located 5 centimeters below the navel, this chakra relates to expression, manifestation, change, creative abilities, feelings and emotions, and sexual and passionate love. It is often called the seat of life.

Location Lower abdomen to navel, the sacral spine
 Color Orange
 Element Water
 Functions Procreation, assimilation of food, desire, sexuality
 Glands Gonads
 Body Parts Genitals, ovaries, testicles,

uterus, spleen, bladder, kidney, large bowel

Gems/Mineral Carnelian, coral, gold calcite, amber, citrine, gold topaz, peach aventurine

Foods Liquids – orange fruits and vegetables

When Balanced

Working harmoniously and creatively with others, generosity, passion for life, surrendering to change, flexibility, genuine intimacy, freedom

When Imbalanced

Over-indulging in food, habits, or sex, sexual and relationship inadequacy, confusion, aimlessness, jealousy, envy, impotence, urinary problems, lower back pain,

embarrassment/shame of body

THIRD CHAKRA: COMPLETION

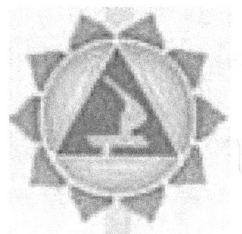

Being committed to achieving something in the world and having the personal power to carry it through underlies the qualities of this chakra. Are you using your will to inspire others or to manipulate them? Choice, action, vitality, power, transformation and will are key to this chakra.

Location Solar Plexus/navel
Color Yellow
Element Fire
Functions Vitalizes the sympathetic nervous system, digestive processes, metabolism, emotions (anger, guilt,

passion)

Glands Pancreas, adrenals

Body Parts Stomach, gallbladder, liver, muscles, nervous system

Gems/Mineral Citrine, gold topaz, amber, tiger, gold calcite, gold

Foods Starches – yellow fruits and vegetables

When Balanced

Empowerment of self and others, leadership qualities, will power, confidence, high self esteem, self control, being responsible, radiance, warmth, transformation, humor, laughter, immortality

When Imbalanced

Low self-worth and confidence, being manipulated by others, low energy, inconsistency, dogmatic conformity, spiritual snobbery

FOURTH CHAKRA: HEART

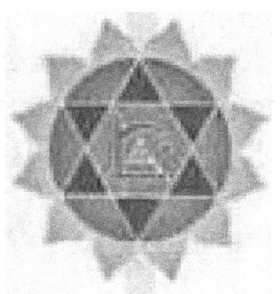

Being motivated by love and joy through accepting that everything is in right Divine order, creates harmony from this energy vortex. It is the mid-point between heaven and earth. It brings about acceptance of oneself and others.

Location Center of the chest, on the sternum
 Color Green
 Element Air
 Functions Anchors the life force from the Higher Self. Energizes the blood and physical body with the life force. Blood

circulation.
Glands Thymus
Body Parts Arms, hands, heart, lungs, circulatory system
Gems/Mineral Emerald, green and pink tourmaline, malachite, green jade, green aventurine, chrysoprase, kunzite, rose quartz, ruby
Foods Green fruits and vegetables
When Balanced

Divine/unconditional love, forgiveness, compassion, understanding, unity, harmonious relationships, seeing God in All, acceptance, peace, openness, contentment, joy, service with ease

When Imbalanced
Repressing love and alienation, emotional instability, grief, loneliness

FIFTH CHAKRA: THROAT

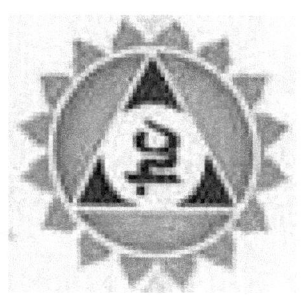

Communication is the focus using mantra and sound. Learning and needing to efficiently express oneself are the main attributes of this truth center.

Location Throat area
 Color Sky blue
 Element Ether
 Functions Speech, sound, vibration, communication, creative expression
 Glands Thyroid, parathyroid
 Body Parts Neck, shoulders, ears, throat, mouth, hypothalamus
 Gems/Mineral Turquoise, chysocolia, celestite, blue topaz, sodalite, lapis luzuli, aquarmarine, azurite, kyanite
 Foods Blue and purple fruits and

vegetables

When Balanced

Power and truth of the spoken word. Hearing what has not been said. Comfortable with the sound of your voice. Best ideas put into action. Integration, truth, knowledge, wisdom, loyalty, honesty, reliability, gentleness, kindness, courage

When Imbalanced

Cunning, shyness, inadequate communication, speech challenges, listening difficulties, ignorance, lack of discernment, frustration

SIXTH CHAKRA: THIRD EYE

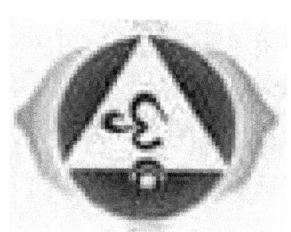

What you expect to see is what is seen — differently, with inner sight, discernment and clarity as you transcend time and duality. It governs clairvoyance, dreams, vision and memory.

Location Center of the forehead, between the eyes through the root of the nose
Color   Indigo/dark   blue
Element   Light
Functions Vitalizes the lower brain (cerebellum) and central nervous system. Vision.
Glands Pituitary (some sources say pineal gland)
Body Parts Left Eye, nose and ears
Gems/Mineral Lapis Lazuli, azurite,

sodalite, quartz crystal, sapphire, indocolite tourmaline
Foods Blue and purple fruits and vegetables

When Being comfortable in any reality, soul Balanced realization, intuition, insight, imagination, clairvoyance, concentration, peace of mind, wisdom, seeing energy within, and beyond, matter and form

When Being out of touch with the body, inability to Imbalanced focus, fear, cynicism, tension, bad dreams, overly detached from the world
SEVENTH CHAKRA: CROWN

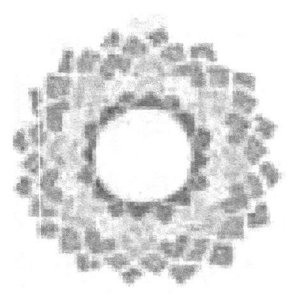

You know the unknown and are conscious of the Infinite. You take abstract ideas and put them into concrete form. The elements of each chakra is located here. It enables the understanding of information, consciousness and awareness.

Location Top center of the head, projecting through the anterior fontanel
Color Violet
Element Thought
Functions Vitalizes the upper brain (cerebrum)
Glands Pineal
Body Parts cerebral cortex, central nervous system, right eye, nervous system
Gems/Mineral Amethyst, alexandrite, diamond, sugilite, purple fluorite, quartz crystal, selenite
Foods Fasting
When Balanced

Higher Self is one with human personality. Spiritual will
When Lack of inspiration Imbalanced

EIGHTH CHAKRA: SOUL STAR

Located about 30 centimeters above the crown of the head, this chakra is the first of the higher chakra system that allows us to make a clear connection to the heart chakra and our soul self. It assists us in realizing Divine will so humans can become free of toxicity caused by guilt and fear.

The following is an important reminder on how unconditional love can create a healthy balanced chakra system. From **Legion of Light**:

Chapter 9: Considering Reiki For Health

Synopsis

Finding out one is suffering from a certain disease can be frightening. Then to be bombarded with a lot of procedures and processors add to the already stressful state. Besides all this, having to choose from the various options available for the treatment of the said health problems can be quite confusing to say the least.

A Mind Opener

When an easy and non invasive option is available, coupled with the possible health recovery tag, most people are keen to explore these avenues of healing. However embarking on the reiki style of treatment, should never be at the expense of discontinuing all other current medications, or other ongoing medical procedures.

Reiki is a holistic style of treatment which is meant at its early stage to compliment any preexisting treatment the patient may be undergoing. The reiki element is meant to work with the positive energy derived to combat any preexisting negatives in the body system. As reiki energy is meant to be dispersed according to the particular area needing the positive energy, prior diagnoses or prescriptions are unnecessary. Besides being unnecessary it is also unethical to make any such recommendations.

People is severe medical conditions have made claims of a certain percentage of success after using reiki as an added and complimenting healing feature. The positive energy emitted from the reiki practitioner unto the recipient is often noted as very calming and helpful. With this positive energy flowing through the recipient's body some of the medically impaired elements can be eradicated to a certain extent. If continued for a longer period of time, if is even possible to eradicate the ailment altogether. For an individual that takes his or her health for granted and does not really take precautions to keep a healthy diet and lifestyle, taking up reiki can be the turning point to a better understanding of the importance of good health and mind conditions.

Chapter 10: The Chakras And The Energy Body

We are all more than just bones, muscles and organs. There is a life force in us, that makes us alive and that gives the fuel to your body so it can get on with its business of living. This life force, which is called prana by the yogis, circulates in your body through meridians, which are lines of energy that go down your body. But the energy itself is drawn into you through your chakra system, which are little vortexes of energy that swirl and suck energy into your aura, that egg shaped bubble that surrounds your physical body. Most eastern traditions agree on these principles and acupuncture and shiatsu, to name only two, are based on these principles of energy.

Circumstances in life, such as illnesses, accidents and traumas, but also mind sets, can create energy blockages in the body that, if left untreated, can in turn create illnesses or malfunctions in the body. Removal of blockages can be done by acupuncture, shiatsu but also by reiki. Reiki is an energy that clears blockages and helps the system spin at the rate that it is supposed to. It is non-intrusive and very gentle and can be given to anyone of any age, babies, pregnant women and the elderly, and also to animals and plants. Old people and babies benefit particularly from receiving reiki. Reiki is wonderful during pregnancy. The reason I recommend it for mums to be is that it makes you aware of very subtle levels of energy and can help calm a baby after they are born, but even from when they are In the womb.

We have seven main chakras in our bodies. Again, yogis and Tibetans have given them each a name. Chakras are said to be spinning vortexes of energy and when they are balanced and functioning well, they spin clock wise at the front of our bodies and anti-clockwise in our backs, drawing in energy from the nature and our environment. When we are unbalanced however, these chakras can spin very slowly or even be blocked or spin counter clockwise. In that case, the area that they govern is deprived of vital energy and if the problem is not resolved, it can lead in time to illnesses or malfunction of the organs of that region.

A traditional colour has been associated with each chakra (see diagram above) and together they form the colours of the rainbow. However, not everyone complies with this scheme. And evolution can bring some changes in the colour scheme.

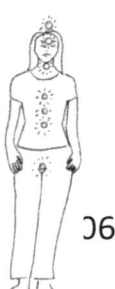

We have numerous other chakras that are smaller. The most important of those minor ones are the ones in our hands, knees and feet. The hand chakras are usually used to pour energy out, hence the hands of light or healing hands. The knees are important for progression and the feet are essential for grounding and drawing energy from the earth, but also for getting rid of negativity, a bit like a plug in a bathtub that needs to be open when cleaned.

7 - Crown chakra: purple or silver colour, the portal to other dimensions, particularly spiritual dimensions. It governs the pineal glands.

6 - Brow or third eye chakra: indigo colour, seat of clairvoyance and clear vision, links to ears. Energy of clarity and compassion. It governs the eyes and pituary glands.

5 - Throat chakra: sky blue colour, seat of clairaudience, clear speech and integrity. Energy of right speech and truth. It governs the thyroid, the ears, the throat and voice.

4 - Heart chakra: green and pink colour, seat of the emotions. Energy of compassion. It governs the heart, lungs and thymus.

3 - Solar plexus chakra: yellow, seat of self confidence and interaction with others. Energy of endurance. It governs the spleen, liver, gall bladder, stomach, Pancreas and adrenals.

2 - Naval chakra: orange colour, links with desires and one to one relationships. Energy of survival and desire. It governs the genitals, the reproductive organs, bladder, prostate, the Lymphatic system and adrenals.

1 - Base chakra: red colour, seat of survival instinct, connects to mother and earth energy, base of the kundalini. Energy of manifestation. If unbalanced, can lead to inability to find a home or be part of a community. It governs the gonads, pelvis, hips, lower back, sciatic nerve, knees, bowel movements and ovaries.

This is just an introduction and you can find many good books about the energy body. I would recommend the work of **Barbara Brennan, hands of light**, and **Caroline Myss, Energy Medicine** if you want to read more on the subject.

During my classes, I like to teach people to see the aura. The aura is a bubble of energy that protects us and keeps a bubble of protection around us. Most people's auras are very thin as their energy levels are low. In sick people, they can even be almost inexistent. Some people who have had serious traumas can have holes in their auras. That is the reason it is important at the end of a session to smooth the aura to repair it. More of this in Chapter 13.

It is actually relatively easy to see auras, but not necessary. However, I encourage you to try this exercise as it will make you aware of the energy around us. If you want to practice on yourself, place one of your hands in natural light above a sheet of white paper. Look at it without focusing on it. Relax your eyes and loosen the focus so that you are aware of your hand but can't see the details. After a few seconds, you should see like a luminous shadow around your hand.

If you want to practice on another person, place them in front of a wall in neutral colour, again, in natural lighting. Look at them but focus in the distance. After a few seconds, you should start to see a luminous shadow above their head and shoulders. This shadow can be lopsided. It can be white or colourful. Enjoy what you see without trying to analyse.

Practising to see the aura can be very tiring so practice often but for very short periods of time.

Chapter 11: The Fourth Chakra

The fourth chakra is called the anahata in Sanskrit. It is mainly associated with the element of air, and is located in the heart. Recall that the first three chakras teach all individuals of the importance of letting go of fear, guilt, and shame, before embracing strength, creativity, and power. The fourth chakra or air chakra focuses on the concept of unconditional love, and is blocked by the emotion of grief and loss.

More about the air chakra

If you were successfully able to open your first three chakras, then cleansing your fourth chakra will be easy. The air chakra is important because it serves as the bridge between your mainly physical chakras, and your mainly spiritual and mental chakras. It is the chakra that deals heavily with love, and your most intimate relationships.

Do you remember your first heartbreak? What did it feel like? Do you recall a tightening of the chest, a pain that most people would describe as though someone or something was pulling part of their away? This is a physical sign that the fourth chakra is suffering imbalance. Why? What does it take for the air chakra to be in balance anyway? Isn't unconditional love too idealistic a standard for a chakra's balance?

The most important thing you have to understand about love is this: you cannot ever hope to give someone unconditional love if you do not first love yourself. The fourth chakra teaches that love is a gift that is already inside us, simply waiting to be given to others so that a cycle of love and understanding may ensue. While understanding what unconditional love is will certainly be difficult, it is not something you should grieve or worry over. Instead, you should rejoice in the concept of unconditional love, and trust that you too, will soon have the ability to give and receive such pure, powerful energy.

Opening the air chakra

Follow the steps below to open, cleanse or recharge your fourth chakra.

Step 1: Sit in an open space that is devoid of any noise or distractions.

Step 2: Close your eyes, breathe deeply, and feel the air that surrounds you. Feel it envelop you with a loving, reassuring presence.

Step 3: Think about all the things that have caused you grief. Lay these thoughts out before yourself as honestly as you can.

Step 4: Now think about love. Have you ever doubted love? Have you been in a relationship where you feel as if your love was wasted, discounted? Have you ever been afraid to love, afraid to get hurt because of love? Have you ever doubted the love of a special person for you? Think about them; lay them out before yourself as you have with your grief.

Step 5: Slowly, slowly release all your grief and doubts about love. Let the air, that is evaporated water, thinner earth, and the partner of fire, blow all of your grief, pain and doubt away. Let the air fill you with refreshing energy, calm and reassuring energy. Let the wind cleanse and recharge your fourth chakra as you let go of your grief, and come to understand that these things are part of life, and play an important role in your growth.

The air chakra can also be strengthened by associating wearing clothes or eating food that is of the color green. Spinach, broccoli and kale and celery are good greens to eat for emotional healing.

Chapter 12: Circles Meditation

Get into a comfortable position. Allow yourself to begin to follow your breath, eyelids joining, allowing thoughts and feelings to drift through your mind. Just allow yourself to observe and follow the in breath and the out breath. Attune to your receptive nature with each in breath, attune to letting go and give out into the world with each out breath.

Allow a wave of relaxation to pass throughout your body (you can mention specific body parts here) Receive healing and love on the in breath, and let go of what you do not need on the out breath.

Now feel a light, expansiveness to your being. Focus your breathing on your heart, allowing a softening with each in breath and a sense of your love and connectedness with each out breath. Now allow awareness to focus on the other people in this room. Imagine what it would be like to stand with them, hand in hand, in a large circle.

Find the hand of the person next to you and feel what it is like to take this being into your awareness. Breathe them into your heart. Feel the sense of connection our hands allow us to experience connectedness. Breathe the sense of this group, this circle of beings, deep into your heart.

Now imagine, just beyond the circle of beings in this room another circle. This one of all our beloved ones. Just notice who is here and see them all standing hand in hand embracing our circle. Breathe them into your heart, and breathe out the gift of your awareness to them.

And just beyond this circle, see another circle of ancient Reiki masters, wise ones, teachers - beings who have stood in circles throughout the ages celebrating the blend of life. See them standing hand in hand. See another circle of beings of light, angels beyond them. Breathe them into your awareness and breathe out the gift of your love and recognition to all of them.

And one more circle - in this one, imagine the other beings who share the planet with us - the ones who fly in the air, the ones who swim in the sea, and the four-legged ones. See them all standing paw in wing, side by side, embracing the circle of the ancient ones, embracing the beloved ones, embracing us.

Feel us all standing connected on our precious planet sending her the gift of our love and recognition. Breathing in the gift of connection and oneness. Take all of this into your hearts. Pause a while.

Gently allow your awareness to return to your own breathing. Let go of the hands in yours. Breathe into your centre. Allow yourself to slowly return to full consciousness and open eyes.

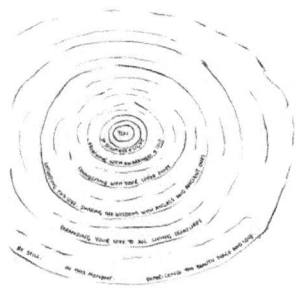

Another suggested meditation

Crystal Cave

Settle yourself comfortably. Allow your eyes to gently close. Become aware of your breath, as your breathing slows and quietens.

Picture yourself at the mouth of a cave. The cave is almost transparent, as though made of ice. It is a crystal cave. Feel your feet on the ground - then walk into the cave. It opens up into a fantastic cavern, which glistens and sparkles as though lit by an invisible light. You gaze at it, stunned by its wonder and beauty. A tinkling music fills the cave, like wind-chimes. You walk deeper and deeper into the crystal cave, hearing your footsteps echo in the hollow cavern. Ahead, a brilliant white light is shining, at the opening to a passageway. You walk towards it and enter the passageway - and find yourself in another crystalline cavern, dazzling in its magnificence.

In the centre of the cavern is a small crystal column, on which a golden chalice stands. The chalice glistens in the light. This is the Chalice of Abundance, placed there by you Higher Self. It is full to the brim of a wondrous liquid, which will bring abundance into your life. As you hold the Chalice, become aware of any resistance you might have to drinking from it. (What are your thoughts and feelings? What are your fears?) Then see your resistance become bubbles, which float away into the cavern, burst and are gone. When you are ready, drink from the Chalice. Drink and drink - for were you to drink a whole ocean, the Chalice would still be full to the brim. There is enough abundance here for all to share. This is not simply wealth of possessions but of happiness, contentment and fulfillment too.

If you have specific needs or desires, then throw a symbol into the chalice, and watch it multiply by the thousand, until it overflows the Chalice and floods out onto the floor of the cavern. If you desire more love in your life, throw a tiny heart into the Chalice - and see the chalice become filled with tiny hearts, which pour out over the crystal column. If you want more success at work, toss a star into the Chalice, and it will brim with tiny stars. If you want more money, toss in a gold coin and you will quickly be ankle-deep in gold.

(Note any fears or uneasiness you might feel as the Chalice gives you what you desire. Breathe deeply and allow these fears to dissipate.)

When you have finished, replace the Chalice - and thank your Higher Self for providing its abundance. Know that you can return to the Chalice at any time.

Then gently again become aware of your breath. Feel your feet, hands and body. Come back to full consciousness and open your eyes to the room.

Chapter 13: Hands On Healing" In Religion

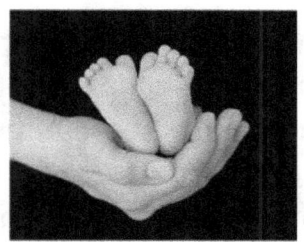

Synopsis

The laying on of hands is a religious ceremony that goes with particular religious practices, which are encountered throughout the world in variable forms.

Laying On Of Hands

n Christian churches, this practice is utilized as both a symbolic and formal technique of invoking the Holy Spirit mainly during baptisms and confirmations, healing services, blessings, and ordination of priests, pastors, elders, deacons, and additional church officers, along with a assortment of additional church sacraments and holy observances.

The laying on of hands was a behavior referred to on a lot of occasions in the Tanakh to accompany the conferring of a blessing or authority. For instance, Isaac blessed his son Jacob by laying on of hands found in Genesis 27:27.

Moses appointed Joshua with semikhah - i.e. by the laying on of hands: Num 27:15-23, Deut 34:9. The Bible adds that Joshua was thereby "filled with the spirit of wisdom". Moses likewise appointed the seventy elders (Num 11:16-25). The elders later appointed their successors in that way. Their successors successively appointed other people. This chain of hands-on semikhah carried on through the time of the Second Temple, to an unresolved time. The precise date that the original semikhah succession ended isn't clear. A lot of medieval authorities trusted that this happened during the reign of Hillel II, around the year 360 CE. Even so, it appears to have carried on at least until 425, when Theodosius II executed Gamaliel VI and stifled the Patriarchate and Sanhedrin.

Aaron and the High Priests who came after him symbolically transferred the sins of the Children of Israel to a sacrificial goat by the laying on of hands: Leviticus16:21.

In the New Testament the laying on of hands was affiliated with the welcoming of the Holy Spirit as in Acts 8:14-19. At first the Apostles laid hands on new believers as well as believers.. In the early church, the use continued and is still utilized in a wide assortment of church ceremonies, like during confirmation.

The laying on of hands, called "the Royal Touch" or "the Divine Touch," was executed by kings in England and France, and was believed to heal scrofula (also known as "King's Evil" at the time), a name devoted to a number of skin disorders. The rite of the king's touch started in France with Robert II the Pious, but legend later ascribed the practice to Clovis as Merovingian father of the Holy Roman kingdom, and Edward the Confessor in England. The belief carried on to be common throughout the Middle Ages however started to die off with the Enlightenment. Queen Anne was the last British monarch to claim to have this divine power, though the Jacobite pretenders likewise claimed to do so. The French monarchy carried on to believe and perform the act up till the French Revolution. The act was typically performed at big ceremonies, frequently at Easter or additional holy days..

Chapter 14: Additional Healing Techniques (Advanced Students Only)

This chapter contains additional healing techniques, which are taken from various Reiki and healing schools. It is up to you whether you try them. This is aimed at Advanced students, and for reference and background knowledge.

DISTANT HEALING

It is important that you learn this technique through a professional Reiki course.

Distant healing and symbols are part of many Reiki schools, including the traditional Usui school, but there are variations on distant healing techniques and additional symbols, including:

The traditional Reiki technique for distance healing is done through an object, such as a teddy bear.

It could also be done with prayer and intention.

In Blue Star Celestial Energy, distant healing is done by the method of Exomatosis (out of body experience).

A technique from Spirituality (UK): imagine your hands cupped, holding a great mound of sparkling dust. Imagine yourself blowing into sparkling magic dust and dust disseminates itself around whole world, reaching out to all who need healing. Blow on dust with loving heart and see your loving heart reach out to four corners of the earth.

Thigh and knee method: Imagine your right knee is the person's head, right mid-thigh is their body and the rest of your right tight is their legs and feet. Your left knee is the back of their head, your left mid-thigh is their back and the rest of your left thigh is the back of their legs and feet.

Using a photograph.

Writing their name of a piece of paper. This can also include a Reiki Box, where you continually put pieces of paper of people and situations e.g. war, in the box once a week or when needed (you remove the paper later). You can also keep crystals in the box to aid healing.

From Angel Healing, imagine that person surrounding by beautiful loving light from the Angels (pink for love, blue for protection, white for healing).

In Kundalini Reiki, it is done by visualising a name or person in your hands, then placing your hands in prayer position to heal that person. You can also use this technique to heal situations, past lives, the trauma of birth or the past, our DNA (diseases) or crystal deposits within your body (Crystalline Reiki). They recommend healing yourself before beginning to heal others.

Timeline Reiki: The future or past e.g. war zones, places of mourning or great trauma, your own personal trauma, job interview in the future, child birth if you or someone else is pregnant, etc. You can also combine Timeline Reiki for key events with other therapies such as NLP or Hypnosis if for yourself, as well as Reiki symbols.

When doing a Distant Healing, make sure you (1) ask for protection for both yourself and the person; (2) that they only receive it if they want to receive it – if not may it go to someone else or an event that is of benefit; (3) it is only for their highest good; and (4) that receive it when it is safe, e.g. when they're lying down in bed (rather than driving or any activity that needs concentration).

USING SYMBOLS

When you are using a symbol, you are channeling a source of healing and love. Using a symbol could be compared to ringing a telephone number. This can all be interpreted according to your own beliefs. If using a symbol from a certain religion, this is not the same as attending or following a religious school, which has it owns ethics and traditions. You are just healing.

The traditional Usui school uses four symbols, although it is said that Usui only used three (it may have been added in the Hayashi-Takata lineage where symbols where more important). The Usui symbols are introduced at level two as power (Cho Ku Rei), mental emotional (Sei Hei Kei) and distance healing (Hon Sha Ze Sho Nen).

Master level three introduces the final master symbol (Dai Ko Myo).

In Usui, the Reiki Mental Sandwich can be used in many different ways to release imbalances e.g. additions, bad habits, trauma, unhealthy beliefs and feelings. This is done through Power, Emotional/Mental, Power. The Complete Reiki Sandwich in Usui is Power, Emotion/Mental, Power, Hon Sha Ze Sho Nen, Power.

There are many symbols associated with different schools of Reiki. I would recommend learning these through a professional Reiki course. For example, the additional master symbol of Dumo, both as a masculine and feminine version. An anti-clockwise symbol for power Cho Ku Rei, which is said to be matter to spirit (rather than the clockwise spirit to matter). Celti Reiki has a lot of symbols that look similar to runes. There is an angel wings infinity symbol. A symbol of a cross for Christianity or Jesus. The Om symbol used in Buddhism or Hinduism. More recently the Double Helix symbol used in DNA Reiki. And so on.

When using sacred symbols, always make sure through ethics, prayer and intention that it is only for the highest good. Always choose symbols that are associated with love and positivity.

Personally, if you know many different symbols from different schools, don't try to use them all at once as the Reiki will be too open and unfocused.

Reiki and other forms of healing can equally be sent just through intention and prayer, without symbols. Spiritual Healing does not use any symbols. Do what works best for you, symbols or no symbols.

ANIMAL AND PLANT HEALING

You can also heal animals (or plants!).

Always make sure that both you and the animal are safe. As with humans, always get the permission of the animal (you can't ask them, but if they wriggle or run off, then stop). You could also do this as a distance healing exercise (if you are trained).

- Simply, do a dedication at the beginning of the Reiki (as with humans, to protect you both).

- Place your hands on or close to the animal (e.g. head, body), and channel healing.

- Close down afterwards. Make sure you're animal is safe.

ANGEL HEALING

This is the same principle as regular Reiki or healing, except you are channelling Angels and Angelic energy.

Get permission of the person you are healing, and tell them it is "Angel" Healing. It is still best to say prayers to yourself quietly, rather than out loud.

Say a prayer and dedication at the start of the healing, but dedicate it only to Angels. In your prayer, include both your Guardian Angel, and your client's Guardian Angel. You can also include Archangels, if you wish. Say that you ONLY wish to work with Angel energy.

Ask Archangel Michael to protect you, as you still need to protect yourself and your client as you are opening up to different energies.

Channel healing as you would normally, focusing on different parts of the body. Either do this intuitively or follow a sequence of hand movements (e.g. start on shoulders, 7 chakras, finish on head).

When you are ready, finish healing and close down. Say thank you to the Angels and ask them in prayer to help you close down and finish the healing.

TYPES OF ANGELS

- Archangels and other senior or higher level Angels e.g. Archangel Michael for protection.

- Guardian Angel – Personal Angel.

- Angels for specific purposes – e.g. Angel of your house; the Ocean; travel; work etc.

- Solar Angels (in Tibetan Reiki) – Angels of Energy.

To learn more about Angels and Angel Healing see Diana Cooper (School of Healing), Doreen Virtue (Angel Therapy Practitioner ATP), Angel Flames Reiki, Angel Reiki, Archangel Seichim, Stephen Lovering's Colours of Angels, and Sapphires of Angels, amongst others.

DNA REIKI

More recently, a new tradition of Reiki has emerged called DNA Reiki. This uses the Double Helix symbol and it said to heal at a deeper level to include changes to a person's DNA. This is dependent upon what you belief and there could be a debate that Reiki has its own intelligence and unlimited power. However I feel there is no harm in adding the DNA Double Helix symbol to your practice e.g. on your hands or on the client.

REIKI SHARES

These are also called Reiki Circles or Reiki Groups. It is where qualified Reiki healers come together as a group to practice on each other (Reiki level 1 or above). This is for training purposes, and to each enjoy and receive Reiki. It can also be social. It is also good for sending out distant healing and prayers as a group.

It can done on a chair, or lying down. The person lying down (or sitting) will have more than one person giving them hands on healing at the same time, i.e. you'll have 2, 3 or more pairs of hands on you! It can be a very intense healing experience.

This is also a Japanese Reiki technique (Shu Chu-Reiki and Reiki Mawashi techniques).

The Spiritual Church (UK) also does multiple healing in the same way. It is worth noting, that the Spiritual Church also teach healing over 18 months to 2 years because they believe that a lot more practical time is needed to learn to how to heal properly and responsibly. I think that Reiki Shares are a perfect way of achieving this, as they offer additional training and practice to the official Reiki courses available. It is a good idea to allow a few months between each level of Reiki training and attunement.

Make sure you go to a Reiki Share that is being run by a good teacher who has proper training and experience. There are plenty of Reiki Shares out there if you are unsure.

CHAKRA HEALING USING COLOUR AND VISUALISATION

This technique helps to balance and heal your chakras through visualisation and colour.

Set aside some time. (beginners start with a small amount of time e.g. 5-10 minutes).

Remove distractions (turn off phone, TV etc).

Sit in a comfortable position, making sure your spine is straight at all times. E.g. sit crossed legged, in a chair, or lie down.

Breathe in and out naturally with your diaphragm. In and out through your nose.

Imagine pure white healing light going into your crown chakra and filling the whole of your body.

Focus on each of your 7 chakras, one by one, visualising them in your mind.

Start with your crown chakra. Do you notice or feel any imbalance? Does it feel strong? Weak? Repeat this with all of your other chakras.

Go back to the chakras that felt like they needed healing. One by one, visualise colour and/or healing going into them and around them. For example, the base chakra is healed by the colour red.

Repeat this until you feel like all your chakras have been balanced and healed.

Imagine the pure white light going into the ground. Put a protective cloak or bubble around you. Wiggle your fingers and toes, and slowly start to come round and finish the session.

GATEWAY CHAKRA HEALING

This is used in the Radiance Technique – 7th level.

Put one hand on the crown chakra and one on the gateway chakra (in the air above crown chakra). Channel Reiki for several minutes.

Put one hand on the third eye chakra and one on the gateway chakra (in the air above crown chakra). Channel Reiki for several minutes.

Put one hand on the crown chakra and one on third eye chakra. Channel Reiki for several minutes.

CRYSTALS

Some people like to use crystals in their healing room, in a grid, during their practice or directly onto their patient (chakras or problem area),. As always, this depends on your client. Common crystals include: -

- Rose Quartz (for love),

- Amethyst (positive transformation and spiritual growth),

- Azurite (self confidence and creativity),

- Citrine (abundance),

- Ruby (passion),

- Selenite (peace),

- Tigers Eye (clarity and balancing emotions),

- Fluorite (protection and cleansing),

- Jade (soothing),

- Sapphire (energy and mental stability),

- Clear Quartz (master – you can use for anything).

AFFIRMATIONS

This is saying a positive statement to yourself, quietly or out loud. This helps you mentally and emotionally (similar to Cognitive Behaviour Therapy). Some people believe that it also helps you spiritually – you attract what you send out.

Affirmations have to be positive. For example, you cannot say, "I am NOT poorly", instead say "I AM healthy". Believe it when you say it.

You can say these in meditation or in your everyday life (e.g. when driving, going for a walk, washing up). Some people also like to say them in private, in front of a mirror as they feel that it is very powerful (although, it can be painful at first). It might be best to say them to yourself, quietly in your head, but you can say them out loud if it is appropriate and there's no-one around.

This is also used as part of one of the Japanese Reiki Techniques called Nentatsu-Ho (which can be learnt on a course, or buy a good book).

- I AM healthy.
- I AM loved.
- I AM confident.
- I have successful, healthy relationships.
- I AM patience.
- I AM / FEEL peaceful and calm.
- My heart is filled with love and peace.
- I AM compassionate and tolerant.
- I have a positive healthy love life.
- I attract positive people in my life.

- I AM beautiful.

- I HAVE healthy self-esteem.

- I have a positive healthy self-image.

- I LOVE myself.

RELEASING EMOTIONS

Healer, heal thyself!

Let go of your negative emotions or thoughts by trying some of the following:

- Write down thoughts, feelings and emotions on a piece of paper. Be as angry, irrational and emotional as you like. MAKE SURE NO ONE SEES IT – when you've finished, tear it up, shred it, throw it away in a safe place.

- You could also do this as a letter to a person who you have unresolved issues with.
DON'T SEND IT AND MAKE SURE NO ONE

SEES IT – when you've finished tear it up, shred it, throw it away in a safe place.

- Of course, sometimes it is appropriate to talk to a person directly if you have any issues in your relationship that you wish to resolve. You could also try some of these techniques first so that you are clear what your problems and feelings are beforehand.

- Do something creative - art, music, writing, poetry. Release your emotions expressively. Be as childish and playful as you like. It is the process that matters, not the end result.

- Tell a friend about your problems for support and advice is always good. Just respect that they may have problems themselves.

- Sometimes you need professional advice such as a counselor or therapist.

- If you are angry about something, (and it's safe for yourself and others), try punching your pillow or punch bag to release anger. Make sure both you and others are safe. Don't hurt or strain your wrists and hands.

- If you are angry or upset about something or someone, imagine speaking to that person about it. What do you want to say? What is the outcome you would like? Deep down, what are you really upset about? Remember to send them loving thoughts and healing afterwards (as well as yourself).

- Go for a gentle walk or brisk run.

- If you have a lot of pent up anger, maybe go to a field in the middle of nowhere, or empty house and try shouting really loud "aaaggghhhh". Or instead, sit in your car, in a remote area, car engine switched OFF, windows up, doors shut, "aaarrrggghhh." These work really well.

However, I would be extremely cautious as you want to make sure no-one is around, that no-one will be offended or upset, and that you are not trespassing or parked illegally or dangerously. Also, you don't want to be locked up for being crazy!

- If you have any blocked emotions, listen to music or watch a film that helps you to release these emotions e.g. angry song, sad film.

- Some people like to keep a diary to release emotions. Make sure it's in a safe place.

- You can also get hypnotherapy CDS for releasing emotions and improving self-esteem and confidence. For example, Glynn Harrold or Paul McKenna.

- Meditate or do Reiki on yourself!

Repeat these exercises as many times as you like.

Always make sure that you and others are safe. Don't send out the letters.

Send out loving thoughts afterwards.

Chapter 15: Everyday Reiki

Follow the practices mentioned below and you would have successfully harnessed the profound power of Reiki to work for you in everyday life.

Eat Reiki

Learn how to energize your food. Through this way, you'll get Reiki into your body and make sure it reaches every cell that needs it. The idea is to get your food thoroughly charged with the healing energy. When you start to reach for your mouth, the benefits wired into the core of Reiki will permeate your being and enhance its luster from within. To absorb the Reiki healing energy through the food you eat, use the method below, but make sure you explore your creativity.

Place your food in a neat and quiet place, and then fix your gaze at it. Start to form a vivid imagination and outright intention that there is a dense cloud of healing energy like a swathe few feet above the food.

Now start to heighten your consciousness by increased concentration and intent that healing energy starts to nestle like dews on the food, saturating and energizing it with a cluster of light.

In your imagination release the dew and let it flow the more till it becomes a dropping deluge of healing energy.

It's time to draw Cho Ku Rei (end of the session) and usher in the feeling of earnest gratitude.

It's time to forget all other things and enjoy your Reiki-rimmed food.

If you can endeavor to make this technique a consistent practice, it will leave a lot of magic in your physical shape and overall health.

Drink Reiki

Virtually everything in this world can be treated with Reiki so far you can send the energy anywhere at any time. Maximize Reiki by enhancing the quality of drinking water you have is a special way by all means. And don't forget that creativity is allowed as you are not just to follow the technique dogmatically. You can, of course, make your own bit of tweaks to it or just flow according to the dictates of your intuition.

You first need your mind very clear, calm, and free so as to enable the flow of the universal energy as perfect alignment is crucial.

Get a glass or cup of water before you and wrap around it your hands as firmly as you can.

With this setup right before your eyes, begin to envision the Power Symbol, and then repeat its name three solid times with all your concentration.

In your mind's eye, let your visualization grow vivid as you see Reiki energy permeating the water through and through till it takes it to a point of saturation.

Let the Reiki-rimmed water down your throat and let it do wonders in your body system.

Dealing With Anxiety

You can deal with anxiety this way below:

The first procedure is to lie down and allow yourself into a very comfortable state to receive the Reiki touch.

Now take some minutes and raise your awareness as you start to imagine that your palms, clasped to your head from behind, are sending waves upon waves of healing energy into your mind to relieve you of debilitating thoughts and replacing them with serenity, ambiance, and happy muses. Then allow your hands immediately to nestle on your heart the moments you have felt soften in the mind.

Just as you did for your mind, let the same measure of healing and light trickle into your heart space. Imagine as your mind becomes detached, as it let go of all encumbrances—releasing pain, stress, hurt, etc.

Now it is time to gently open your eyes and examine the way your heart and body click.

Use Meditation To Relax

Use the method below to relax and keep away anxiety.

The first thing is that you sit down and maintain a straight back to receive Reiki in this method.

Turn up your imagination and see yourself in a dense halo called the universe with the purest healing Reiki energy. See through as the energies start to permeate the entirety of your body and as your exhale floats upon it avalanche of negativities like rage, frustration, depression, worry and etc.

Let your hands glide before your forehead and cover your eyes. You can be sure it will make you very comfortable.

Drag your hands now to over the stomach, keep it there and then relax.

Other areas in the body, mainly the seven chakras, exist where your hands still need to reach and that will take out all the depression and stress out of your body.

Chapter 16: More Poses For Beginners

There are certain poses which are more helpful to beginners than others, in that they cater for people who are not that flexible, allowing them to feel that they have achieved a lot during their yoga practice, without having damaged the body. If you haven't done any exercise for a long time or you have limited flexibility, then these may be the ideal poses for you to try.

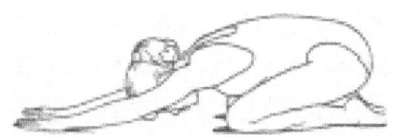

The **Child's Pose** is a particularly good pose to help you to experience the feeling of humility. The reason that it is so good is that you are bowing your head and body down to the floor and one may even imagine this pose being used by servants in days gone by. It's a good pose for helping you to feel more balanced in your life and in a way reminds me of letting go of bad things and being sorry about the negativity in life. It is a very easy pose to achieve and the starting position is a kneeling position with the tops of your feet flat against the carpet. Your feet actually touch and you are encouraged to open your knees before stooping forward and bending to the floor. You can place your head on the floor in front of you and most people can manage this. If you cannot manage it, place a small pillow there to take the weight of your head. This is a great pose, but you need to get the breathing in rhythm with the movements that you make. As such – kneel, breathe in, breathe out and lean forward, breathe in and out while you have your arms stretched out in front of you and your head touches the floor. Breathe in, breathe out, breath in, breathe out and move back to the kneeling position.

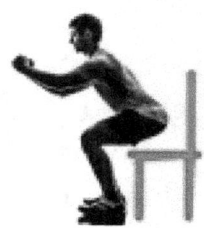

The **chair pose** is another pose that helps you with your posture. If you can imagine that you are about to sit, then you are pretty near this pose, but you need to go through the whole process. Start from a standing position with your feet firmly flat on the floor and touching each other. As you move your body as if you are going to sit down, breathe out and lift your arms up into the air at the same time. Hold that position and breathe in and out. The stance that you are in is very good for posture, but it's great for abdominal region as well. The point is that you need to hold this position just before reaching the sitting position and it is this holding onto the position that works the muscles and helps your upper thigh region as well.

The **Locust pose** is another that helps with flexibility, though you may find it hard to stretch to the limit when doing this. Don't try to. The idea is to do what's comfortable for your body. This exercise helps the waist area but it is also a very good position for people who have jobs at desks and who may have problems with their posture. It will help to get the body back into shape easily. For this exercise you need to be lying on your tummy on the mat. Lie down and relax before you start to do the lifts. Breathe in, breathe out and do this five times. On the last exhale lift the front end of your body and hold your arms out behind you as if you are diving and at the same time, lift the legs from the top of the thigh downward, but make sure that you keep your legs straight.

Basically, what you are doing with this pose is putting all of your weight onto your tummy and stretching the areas that you have lifted. Hold this pose for the count of five and then relax the body. It's important after all exercises to make sure that the body is allowed to relax. As stated previously, this is a great exercise for after the following activities:

- Sitting at a desk all day
- Slouching
- Carrying heavy cases or shopping
- Traveling seated for a long time

Legs up the wall pose is a simple pose that can help circulation and this is especially suited to those who have limited flexibility because it will help to energize the body.

Lie down on your yoga mat and this should be up against the wall. The feet work their way up the wall until the legs are straight, with your bottom against the wall so that your legs are in a straight position against the wall. Some people struggle with this the first time that they try it and if you find that the stretch is too much simply breathe in and move one knee down to your tummy and hug it and then place it back against the wall. Then do the other leg in the same way. For circulatory problems, this is the perfect exercise and those who have been busy all day will really appreciate that feeling that they get from a very relaxing position in yoga.

If you make up a program of yoga exercises, remember, it's not about how many exercises you do. It's about variation to cover the parts of the body that need it and taking it slowly enough to actually achieve good positions and movement that goes in rhythm with your breathing.

That's more important than speed and is something that you need to practice above all else. It's not about how much mobility you have or how hard you push yourself. All yoga exercises are a natural progression and as you get more and more accustomed to using your breath to help you to get into the positions stated, you will find that your ability will also improve.

Chapter 17: Reiki Faqs

How easy is Reiki?

Reiki is easy and is a very simple procedure. Children can also be taught how to perform Reiki. All you need to make sure of is that you are committed to learning.

Is there a certain set of rules for learning and practicing Reiki?

No, there is not. The way you want to learn and begin your practice of Reiki depends on you.

When will I begin feeling the Reiki energy flowing through my body?

When you find a Reiki master, a process called attunement will be performed on you. It is during this time when you will feel the energy flowing through your body, see various lights and colors and feel peace and positivity. Attunement is the process in which the Reiki master prepares your body and initiates it for it to become an effective conduit of energy.

What if I do not feel anything during attunement?

People are different and we feel sensations in different ways. If you do not feel anything during attunement, that is perfectly okay. A Reiki master can successfully perform the attunement process on you even if you do not see or feel anything yet. The energy, lights and colors mentioned earlier are not indications whether the attunement was successful or not.

Do I need to concentrate and redirect my energy to improve the flow of Reiki?

No, you need to let the Reiki flow without exerting any effort on your part. If you wish to perform Reiki on someone and they want you to perform Reiki on them, your intent to heal is all that you need. Just let the Reiki flow naturally from you to make it effective.

If I regularly self-treat, will it be beneficial even if I am just a Reiki beginner?

Yes. Reiki masters started as beginners as well, so there is no need to worry about not getting the benefits just because you are a beginner. If you consistently perform Reiki on yourself, you will be able to restore you body's balance, improve its healing ability and improve your overall well-being.

When should I start performing Reiki on others?

You should only start performing Reiki on others when you are already comfortable with what you are doing and when the process feels natural to you.

Is Reiki beneficial for both the giver and receiver?

Yes. Even if the receiver reaps the mental, physical, spiritual and emotional benefits of Reiki, it is a truly rewarding and gratifying experience for the giver.

Should I feel responsible for a Reiki treatment that has not shown significant results?

The giver should never feel bad about not seeing results, as the healing process relies mainly on the receiver. The receiver should play an active part in his or her own healing process and create certain changes in order for the Reiki to be able to help him or her.

Chapter 18: Living A Kind And Compassionate Life

We have reached the last Reiki principle, "Just for today be kind to all living things".

By this point in our series of Reiki principles you are perhaps noticing the underlying concept – that we are all connected. The new world of quantum physics is opening up deeper understanding of energy and the fact that we are all intrinsically linked.

This principle invites us to look at the concept of being connected – what we do to others we do to ourselves so be kind to all people – and that includes you!

Kindness

Do you consider yourself to be a kind person?

What is kindness?

According to Wikipedia, kindness is "a behaviour marked by ethical characteristics, a pleasant disposition, and concern for others." Another definition is "the quality of being friendly, generous, and considerate".

It is relatively easy to be kind to those whom we love and to those whom we respect. It is not so easy to be kind to those whom we have difficulty with!

However, Usui doesn't say "Be kind to some of the people some of the time" – he says "Be kind to all living things", sometimes translated as "Be kind to all people".

I prefer the "all living things" translation because I feel that we should practice kindness and consideration towards animals and plants and not just other people. I feel we are all connected and therefore kindness should be the foundation upon which we build our lives – it costs nothing to be kind!

So what about these people that perhaps push our buttons – those to whom we find it difficult to practice kindness?

Some teachings say that what irritates us most about someone is often a mirror image of what we don't like about ourselves. This one is a hard one to hear!

For example – if you dislike someone because they are overly critical or judgemental does that mean that perhaps you criticise or judge people too? This is where the previous principle comes into action – do your work honestly. So be honest with yourself – would that be the case?

Sometimes our belief patterns and thinking can get in the way of us being kind. Fear, guilt, resentment and criticism stop us from being kind. These emotions and limiting belief patterns keep us stuck in a negative spiral where we feel like the victim. If you notice that you are in this loop then it is time to break free from it! No more being the victim – switch out the negatives and choose to be more positive.

As I stated right back at the start of this book, we always have a choice in how we think, feel and behave. It is easy to fall prey to victim mentality but that stops you from experiencing the powerful healing benefits of positivity and kindness.

It is time to create a more positive, compassionate and tolerant world don't you think?

It all starts with you!

In the UK we are at a disadvantage because we have been brought up to be reined in and restrained. We find it hard to be positive about ourselves or to express ourselves in a loving way. The British stiff upper lip has a lot to answer for!

Learning to love yourself

Religion has a part to play too. I was brought up in a Christian household and often heard the verse, "Love your neighbour as yourself". I think, however, that the focus was always on the first part of that sentence and the emphasis was to always put others first.

It appeared to be the "Christian thing to do" – to put others first and to love them more than we love ourselves.

That is not what it says though! It says "Love your neighbour as yourself" – in other words as you love yourself. So do you love yourself?

I think this is a concept that we all struggle with, particularly in Northern Ireland. It seems to be a cultural thing to always put yourself down and lift others up. We are pretty useless at accepting compliments and praise - aren't we?

If I asked you to give me a list of all the brilliant things about you, could you do it easily?

For a lot of people it is easier to provide a list of negative things and be really self-critical rather than praise ourselves.

It is almost like we are ashamed of our brilliance. It is seen as "big-headed" to praise yourself or to be proud of your own achievements but why?

We are ALL valuable and we ALL have a role to play.

Each of us is brilliantly unique and we all have our divine inner light to shine. We need to acknowledge how important we are as well as acknowledging and respecting others.

Marianne Williamson writes, in "A Return to Love",

"Our deepest fear is not that we are inadequate. Our deepest fear is that we are powerful beyond measure. It is our light, not our darkness that most frightens us.

We ask ourselves: 'Who am I to be brilliant, gorgeous, talented, or fabulous?'

Actually, who are you not to be? You are a child of God. Your playing small doesn't serve the world. There's nothing enlightened about shrinking so that other people won't feel insecure around you.

We were all meant to shine, as children do. We were born to make manifest the glory of God that is within us. It is not just in some of us – it is in everyone!

And as we let our own light shine, we unconsciously give other people permission to do the same. As we are liberated from our own fear, our presence automatically liberates others!"

I love this quote. It really sums up my beliefs and encompasses what I feel Reiki is all about.

For me, Reiki is about shining your light and thus encouraging others to shine theirs.

I struggled for a long time with loving myself. I felt it was somehow wrong or inappropriate to care deeply for myself. Reiki helped me heal that limiting belief. I began to see that I had a duty of care for myself. I needed to love and respect myself so that I was available to love and respect other people.

I learned that it was important to be nice to myself, to care for my body and mind, to care for my deepest soul desires, to take time out for myself – that I wasn't being selfish at all!

One of my favourite phrases is, "You cannot give from an empty vessel". If you are constantly being kind to everyone else and running about pleasing other people while not taking care of yourself, you will eventually burn out. You will fall apart because you are constantly giving and not receiving – you are out of balance.

I see this all the time in my practice. People will come to me for help with stress, emotional disorders or problems and it usually boils down to the fact that they simply are not taking enough care of themselves.

Having time out for yourself is not selfish – it is a necessity. Looking back to that verse from earlier – we are told to love our neighbour as we love ourselves. So ... if you are not looking after yourself and you do not love yourself in any way then how can you love someone else in the same way? It doesn't make sense does it?

So take the time out — I have learned that I need a lot of time in solitude. I need to give myself the gift of regular walks in nature, good coffee, good books and the precious time to write, paint, meditate or cook in order to feel balanced. Without these things I become stressed and then I cannot help others.

The more you care for yourself, the more you will find that you naturally are more willing to care for others.

If you feel put upon and stressed out by your responsibilities and you are reluctantly "caring" for someone while pushing your needs to the side, you are not actually being kind to them or you! You are acting out of a sense of duty rather than kindness and that is not the same thing at all.

When you begin to give yourself the love, respect, care and attention that you need you increase your happiness factor. This in turn then increases your energy vibration and you have a ripple effect outwards. You begin to have more energy and you want to help others. You learn to say no when it doesn't feel right and learn to say yes when it does.

As you then practice kindness you notice that what goes around comes around! The kinder you are the more you will receive kindness back – particularly to yourself!

The Dalai Lama says,

"When we feel love and kindness towards others, it not only makes others feel loved and cared for but it helps us to develop inner happiness and peace."

Very wise words indeed. So how do we put this into practice?

- Be of service – do something helpful or useful every day for someone. It may be as simple as helping someone lift a heavy bag, donating to a good cause or holding a door open.

- Give affection – we all want to be loved and cared for, so tell the people around you that you love them and you care for them. Hug your partner, your kids and your friends.

- Laugh! Laughter really is the best form of medicine and laughing together is a sure fire way of increasing the vibration in a room. This is the sound of kindness!

- Be grateful – like you have seen before in the Living with Gratitude chapter, write thank you notes, send kind emails and messages, pick up the phone and speak with someone – make an effort to be kind.

● Compliment people – and mean it! Accept compliments when they are given to you – when you reject a compliment it is like throwing a gift back at someone. You are devaluing their opinion and their effort to be kind by rejecting their words, so the next time get a compliment simply say "thank you!"

● Offer a listening ear – how often do you really listen to what is being said. Most of the time when we talk to others, we are thinking about what we are going to say next, rather than listening to them. When you take the time to really listen, you are being kind and compassionate. Often this is all someone needs – someone to listen.

● Take time out for yourself. Make time for solitude and meditation. Make time for walks or long baths. Read your favourite book or magazine. Have a decent cup of coffee and take a break.

Meditation on Loving Kindness

Being kind and compassionate is a beautiful way to be. The more you practice it the more you shine your light and that encourages others to do the same.

It is not always easy but you can work on the difficult people too! Use a meditative practice whereby you visualise being kind to yourself. See yourself smiling at yourself, treating yourself to a gift or walking out in nature.

Next, take the vision outwards and visualise yourself being kind and compassionate to someone you respect – perhaps a teacher or colleague. Feel the warmth of loving kindness emanate from your being and allow it to encompass the other person.

Next, think about someone you love and repeat the process. Feel the warmth rise up and engulf the other person as you visualise love and kindness sweeping over you both.

Finally think about someone you have difficulty with. See yourself smiling at this person and them smiling back. Begin to see their light shine and glow as you offer them love, compassion and kindness.

Working with these meditative techniques and visualisations can really help you deal with difficult people.

Nobody is asking you to be a doormat – always be assertive but always be kind.

Reflect on your positive qualities and reflect on theirs. Begin to see things from a higher perspective and you will notice the changes.

Chapter 19: The 5 Principles Of Reiki

DR. MIKAO USUI NAMED THESE TEACHINGS AS 'The Secret art of Inviting Happiness and The Miraculous Medicine of all Diseases'.

In terms of teaching, Mikao Usui insisted on easy and general methods, nothing lofty. So that Reiki can be easily obtained by anyone.

All the principles here command our subconscious mind to clear negative emotions and build strong positive vibes.

The 5 Principles of Reiki are:

Just for today, do not worry - be happy

Just for today, do not anger - be calm and peaceful

Just for today, do your work honestly

Just for today, be filled with gratitude

Just for today, be kind to every living thing

The Five principles of Reiki are designed to improvise oneself from deep inside, in depth of our hearts we are all imperfect, jealous, mean, lack patience, forgiveness etc. That's why these 5 principles start from "just for today". There is no pressure or stress to work on these principles; you can practice these principles whenever you feel comfortable. **You are not expected to live every moment of your life within the framework of these ideals.**

Just for today, do not worry – be happy

Worry only exists in our mind we have the ability to let it go.

Worrying doesn't take away tomorrows problems, but it will definitely take away today's peace. Worry is created by our fear of puzzling future. Worry is linked to body, mind and spirit. It causes frustration, stress and anxiety that lead to imbalance of the mind and creates health issues. Worry even blocks the root chakra [Muladhara].

Normally we worry about Past or future than present situation. Worrying about your past doesn't change anything we have to learn from the mistakes and move on. When we worry about future, we create a mental pattern to something that hasn't happened yet. We create and experience an emotion before the action.

While worrying we prepare ourselves for the worst possible scenario. This creates an emotion/pattern which gets stored in our aura. Once this negative emotion is established it will be quite tough to see the future in different perspective. Thus, we create the future we are trying to avoid.

As we fear the future, we desire to possess more than what we need to survive. Letting go of worry brings you peace. Peace does not mean to live without challenges; it means we remain peaceful and face challenges of life without worrying.

The best way to overcome worry is to accept life as it is. How you react or take up any problem or situation in your life determines your future. Your thoughts play very important role, if you choose to respond negatively to any problem by getting upset or anxious, you damage yourself. You may even hurt your loved ones through your actions. If you respond positively to any problem considering it as, an opportunity to learn and grow, you will be able to lead happy and fulfilled life.

Take some time and review your life, you feel how little the huge disappointments of the past mean to you now. You may even feel relieved that you didn't receive some of the things you wanted so desperately. Once we start to see life in a broad angle, we realize that the only thing that truly exists is the present moment. So, enjoy, laugh and have fun. Spend some time in a day doing what makes you happy.

Just for today, do not anger - be calm and peaceful

"Holding on to anger is like grasping a hot coal with the intent of throwing it at someone else; you're the one who gets burned" - Buddha.

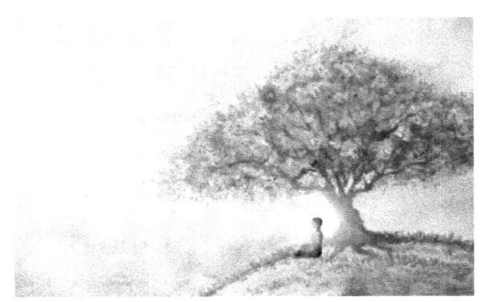

Anger is a reaction, not an action. Anger is an intense emotional response. It is an emotion that involves a strong uncomfortable and aggressive response. Anger can occur when a person feels their personal boundaries are being or are going to be violated. In any argument that leads to anger the person or the situation will have complete power and control over you. Simple realization of what triggers your anger and how you can overcome this destructive emotion allows you to get back control of your emotions. So, you can choose to respond to any situation in positive way instead of negative way.

Anger has 2 destructive ways:

When we don't express and keep it to our self, it affects our physical and mental well-being.

When we try to give it to others, we create negative waves and enforce anger in the opposite person, this way we get negative thoughts which results in bad Karma.

Creating negative energy for any reason will turn out to be harmful to our body, mind and spirit. As we use it much; it becomes part of our thoughts and response system. Which means, instead of considering each situation differently we generalize everything and start using a predetermined response.

When frustrated we create a different perspective of a situation, but anger is our inability to see beyond our predetermined perception. In order to overcome anger, we must change our perception. Instead of keeping it to you or throwing at someone, you can admit it and let go.

Anger burns your positive energy and causes in-digestion. Listen and understand before you respond to any situation. Learn to see from the other person's point of view, break limitations and be broadminded. Meditate everyday it brings peace and calmness automatically. Choose to live a healthier life free from anger.

Just for today, do your work honestly

Be truthful in all aspects of your life.

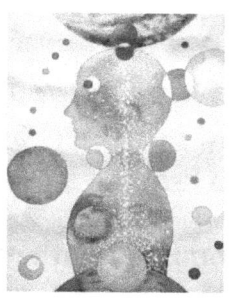

Here work relates to our "life's work". Work on yourself, to develop more love, compassion, peace, happiness, gratitude. Most importantly be true to yourself and be truthful to others.

Honesty is the first chapter in the book of wisdom. Honesty means different things to different people. Being dissatisfied with oneself shows that we are not being honest with ourselves. We feel dissatisfied when we let fear make our choices.

When you are honest to yourself, you do things that make yourself and your family happy; you earning a living without harming others, all these nourishes the soul and brings back balance and harmony to our lives. Love what you do; it keeps you happier and healthier. So that people around you also feel the same.

Just for today, be filled with gratitude

All your needs are already met.

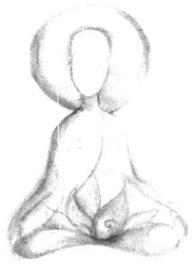

This is an understanding that, just for today, everything we need has been provided. Life gives us what we need to grow and learn in this lifetime instead of what we want. Our present life is just a part of our whole journey. We are here on Earth to pay off our Karmas and gain knowledge through tests. To grow spiritually we have to implement the acquired knowledge.

Gratitude is a selfless act; it can be contagious, in a good way. Gratitude is also a powerful tool for strengthening interpersonal relationships. People who express their gratitude tend to be more willing to forgive others easily. Gratitude promotes better physical and mental health.

Thank yourself for everything you have. Acquiring Materialistic things are necessary to lead an easy life, but acquiring materialistic things more than requirement will also create a bad Karma. Reach out to the needy, be compassionate. Helping others without ego brings abundant joy and compassion to life and keeps you light hearted.

Just for today, be Kind to every living thing

"Kindness is the language the blind can see and the deaf can hear" – Mark Twain

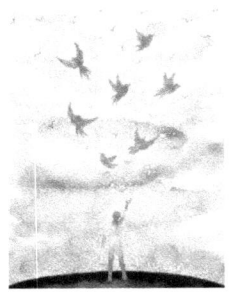

The fifth Principle of Reiki teaches us how to be kind to our-selves first. Also teaches how to mentally tackle any situation with our selves. Kindness is a state of being, it's not an action. One can cultivate kindness by knowing that we are all at different stages on the same spiritual path. We meet each other in many lifetimes, we are all connected. We are here [on Earth] just to learn some Chapter. So, let's be kind and help each other to be good and kind hearted.

Being kind, even in hard times, defines that kindness has become an everlasting part of our life. Being kind doesn't mean that we let others walk over us. Being kind means valuing one's true self and following dharma at the same time. Kindness improves mental well-being and develops respect towards the food we take, the people we meet, animals, trees almost everything around us.

Remember that the Reiki principles are only guidelines for a happy and fulfilling life. The Five principles of Reiki mean different things to each of us. Meditate to unlock the true meaning of each principle and incorporate them into your life. Meditate on these principles every day; it will help to unlock your own perception towards life and transforms life much positively.

Method to meditate on 5 Principles:

Sit comfortably on floor in a quiet place and close your eyes

Do Namaskara/Gassho to calm your mind

Breathe - in naturally, focusing on the point where your two middle fingers meet.

Breath is also referred to the spirit: "prana" [life force] in Sanskrit. Awareness of the breath- breathing in and out nurtures mindfulness. As we focus on breath, inner healing begins and radiates outwards. Let go of all expectations, breathe, relax, focus, center and smile. If your mind keep wandering this physical point helps you to bring back your focus. As you go deep into meditative state you become aware of what's happening inside your mind and body. You may experience different feelings, thoughts and emotions.

Now meditate on 1st principle. [Just for today, do not worry - be happy]

Let it go deep within yourself.

Feel it completely.

Now repeat the meditation on each principle.

At last give thanks to Reiki energy.

Continuously practising this exercise everyday helps you to cultivate pure and healthy mind. This meditation should be practiced on a regular basis. **Recite the Five Principles 2 times a day [Morning and evening].**

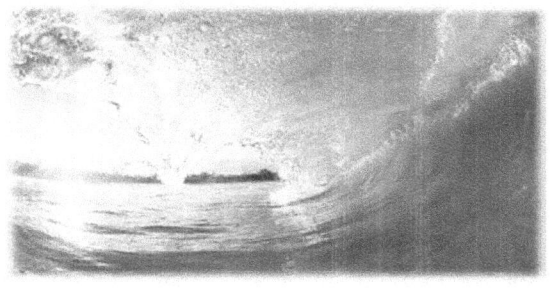

Chapter 20: Explaining Distant Reiki

By Angie Webster

I have written about "Explaining Reiki to Others", but I find that when someone who doesn't know about Reiki wants to know about distant Reiki, it becomes more difficult. Particularly if they want an explanation for how it works. Many people are somewhat able to understand the basic concepts of Reiki in general, but the thought that this could work for someone on the other side of the world can seem too much to take in.

My experience has been that those who are unfamiliar with energy in healing will ask if distant Reiki works through computers, via the internet or over the phone. They have a hard time understanding how a treatment can be sent without connecting it to something tangible for it to flow through that connects both parties.

I admit I was very skeptical of healing energy being real over long distances until I had had several experiences with it. My first experience was in almost 6 years ago. A woman I was friends with was part of a group that met once a week to send healing energies to those in need. She offered to add my name to the list to help me with numerous health problems I had struggled with for years. I said yes, more to humor her than anything. I felt it couldn't hurt because I didn't think it was real.

I was surprised that I could actually feel the energy flow from this group of people each week on the night they met. Even when I forgot about the healing, I would realize I felt peace wash over me and my pain would ease. Within a short time, my health issues began to fade away. I also had more clarity of thought and ability to cope with life.

Yet, even when I learned about Reiki and energy healing, I was still skeptical that it could work. I had seen prayer work from long distances. I believed there also might be special people that could heal from far away. I doubted that anyone could be taught to do it. And I still doubted anyone who said they could do energy work from a distance until they proved it to me.

The telephone, cable TV and Internet all use energy frequencies we can't see in order to function. The electricity in our homes does the same, as does a radio. All of these have to be tuned to the particular frequency they operate at in order to work. They all have ways to adjust the flow of energy built in so that we can turn them on, off or use them in a different way. And all of them were thought too unbelievable to be true when people first heard of them.

Conclusion

I hope this book was able to help you to understand how Reiki can help you achieve a healthy and stress free life. The next step is to seek guidance from a Reiki Master on how you can be attuned and become a Reiki healer, if that is your intention.

Thank you and good luck!

www.ingramcontent.com/pod-product-compliance
Lightning Source LLC
Chambersburg PA
CBHW072004070526
44583CB00015B/1331